non-medical prescribing in health care practice

a toolkit for students and practitioners

edited by

dawn brookes

and

anne smith

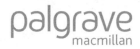

First published 2007 by
PALGRAVE MACMILLAN
Houndmills, Basingstoke, Hampshire RG21 6XS and
175 Fifth Avenue, New York, N.Y. 10010
Companies and representatives throughout the world

PALGRAVE MACMILLAN is the global academic imprint of the Palgrave Macmillan division of St. Martin's Press, LLC and of Palgrave Macmillan Ltd. Macmillan® is a registered trademark in the United States, United Kingdom and other countries. Palgrave is a registered trademark in the European Union and other countries.

ISBN-13: 978–1–4039–9064–8
ISBN-10: 1–4039–9064–6

This book is printed on paper suitable for recycling and made from fully managed and sustained forest sources.

A catalogue record for this book is available from the British Library.

10   9   8   7   6   5   4   3   2   1
16   15   14   13   12   11   10   09   08   07

Printed and bound in China

In memory of our mothers who inspired us and of Jenny Humphries who was a motivational pioneer of nurse prescribing from its inception

Contents

Foreword

The continuing development of non-medical prescribing is a welcome aspect of the modern NHS. Not only does it improve patient care by facilitating access to medicine via the immediate health care team; it also empowers the healthcare professional and ensures efficiency in practice.

As its benefits become firmly established, it is clear that prescribing is not only here to stay, but likely to become even more fundamental to the work of the non-medical practitioner in future. There is, therefore, a growing need for clear and instructive books on the subject, offering insights into new initiatives as well as the overarching policy framework. *Non-Medical Prescribing in Health care Practice* fills that gap, and consequently it should be recommended reading for all of those involved in this field.

Changes to roles and responsibilities provide numerous challenges but similarly their own set of rewards. It is my hope that nurses and allied health professionals will embrace this new era of prescribing with the confidence and enthusiasm it deserves.

LADY CUMBERLEGE

Preface

The aim of this book is to assist those who need to know or would like to know more about non-medical prescribing. This area of practice has been subject to many changes since its inception, particularly recently when the most radical change has been implemented opening the whole formulary to some non-medical prescribers. This text is unique in that it has been written by many different practitioners from a variety of backgrounds who are involved or are likely to be involved in this type of prescribing. There is much to be said about the topic and this book aims to give a taste of how it works in practice.

Non-medical prescribing is a skill that practitioners need to constantly develop during and after prescribing qualifications are obtained. By following some of the guidance in this book and by applying the principles to practice, practitioners can develop their prescribing knowledge with the help of this text. Students will benefit by working through the exercises given throughout the text and by studying some of the underlying principles of prescribing outlined in the different chapters. Qualified prescribers will benefit by gleaning information and the exercises will help with continuing professional development and maintaining competency. There is something for everyone in the text. Managers can see how prescribing has been implemented throughout various settings in the United Kingdom. Doctors, nurses and allied health professionals can read from the perspective of their own individual disciplines. They will also gain a better understanding of the application of prescribing by other health care professionals.

The patient perspective is included, highlighting the high levels of satisfaction gained when they are treated by the most appropriate professional. Patient choice is enhanced by non-medical prescribing and this is demonstrated throughout this book. At the time of writing this is the most up-to-date text on the subject since the major policy changes occurring in May 2006.

The book has been divided into parts in order to assist the reader to navigate through the relevant sections. Exercises and practical case studies are included throughout, helping the reader to pause and reflect on the topics, promoting active learning. This is an innovative text focusing on an area of practice that is enabling practitioners to expand their roles and improve the patient experience.

Acknowledgements

The editors would like to thank the chapter authors for the time given in contributing to this book. We would particularly like to thank Molly Courtenay and Matt Griffiths for taking time out of their busy schedules for their contributions. A special thank you to patients, past, present and future, who make our work and efforts worthwhile and who, we hope, will ultimately benefit. Finally, our thanks go to Palgrave Macmillan, who were prepared to trust in us to produce this book.

Dawn would like to thank her good friends Sue and Ruth for their support and encouragement from the start to the finish of the product. Thank you to my 'adopted' children Susie and Shona who understandingly exclaimed that they were 'book orphans' on a number of occasions!! Thanks also must go to work colleagues for putting up with me when I was distracted. Finally my thanks go to Anne, my co editor, who has maintained the balance in this book.

Anne would like to thank her long suffering family for their tolerance. Also she would like to thank her friends and colleagues who have offered encouragement and support, particularly Kirsten, who could always be relied upon to offer a fresh perspective when inspiration dried up. The most heartfelt thanks go to my co-editor Dawn who has worked tirelessly towards the completion of this project.

Disclaimer

The editors make no claims that the drug dosages in this book are correct. Readers must check the product information and clinical procedures with up-to-date data sheets and clinical guidance and the most recent codes of professional conduct and safety regulations. The editors, authors and publishers do not accept responsibility for any errors in the text. The editors express that the views and opinions in this book are not necessarily their own.

Copyright
Every effort has been made to obtain necessary permission with reference to copyright material. The publisher and authors apologise it, inadvertently, any sources remain unacknowledged and will be glad to make the necessary arrangements at the earliest opportunity.

Notes on contributors

Angela Alexander, BP, MSc, PhD
Angela Alexander qualified as a Bachelor of Pharmacy in 1973 from the University of Bath. She has worked in hospital pharmacy, community pharmacy and academia. She obtained an MSc and a PhD from the University of Aston and a further MSc in Educational and Social Research Methods from the Open University.

In June 2005 she was appointed as Senior Clinical Lecturer at the School of Pharmacy, University of Reading, where she is also a visiting fellow in the Department of Health and Social Care. Angela undertakes contract work in pharmacy practice, education and research.

Diane Birkinshaw
Diane obtained a Diploma in Podiatric Medicine from The Chelsea School of Podiatry in 1986. Her career began in Camberwell Health Authority where she gained experience working with acute and chronic foot conditions. From 1990 she worked for the Podiatry Service West of Berkshire being based at the Royal Berkshire Hospital and helped to develop treatments for patients with major foot complications. Latterly she has moved into a role as Podiatry Education Lead for the service. This role enables her to pass on experiences to students and other health care professionals and contribute to developing the service through education for colleagues and patients.

Mike Brownsell
After working as a charge nurse in Orthopaedic Trauma, Spinal Injury, and Accident and Emergency, Mike was an IV specialist Nurse and then moved to nurse management before entering full time into education. Now Senior Lecturer at the University of Chester, Mike has had an increasing focus on

non-medical prescribing preparation, interprofessional education and the pedagogy of e-learning.

All these interests combined when he had the chance in 2004 to lead a collaborative project involving nine northwest universities to develop blended learning materials for an interprofessional non-medical prescribing programme. The completed materials are now being piloted in the region and recently won an IVCA gold award for 'best internal multimedia computer based programme to train, inform, or educate people'. Having recently embarked on PhD studies into the same area, he now comes with a health warning, if met at a social function.

Josie Cameron

Josie qualified as a therapy radiographer in 1990 and has worked at the Western General Hospital in Edinburgh since then. In 2002, she became one of the first Clinical Radiographer Specialists in Scotland, specialising in breast cancer. Her role was developed to ensure continuity of care and support throughout the patient journey. She is lead practitioner in the simulation of breast cancer patients and also the review clinics, where she has individual weekly consultations with the patients during their radiotherapy treatment to offer advice and support.

Josie's special interests lie in the holistic approach to patient care and she is a qualified aromatherapist and reflexologist. Publications include two case studies in an aromatherapy journal and a paper on radiographer review clinics in the *Journal of Radiotherapy in Practice*.

Molly Courtenay, PhD, MSc, BSc, Cert Ed, RNT, RN

Molly is a qualified nurse with a background in Intensive Care and General Medicine. During recent years she has worked within nurse education and is presently Reader at Reading University. Molly's main research interest is prescribing and medicines management. She has undertaken a number of studies in this area including research for the Department of Health. Her current work includes nurse prescribing in dermatology, diabetes and paediatrics. Molly has produced many publications (including five books). She is currently on secondment to the Royal College of Nursing as their Joint Prescribing Adviser. Molly has recently been made a 'Chair' at the University of Reading and is now a professor.

Helen Crawley, BMBCh, DCH, DRCOG, MRCGP, DFFP
Helen works as a part-time GP, GP trainer, visiting lecturer at the University of Reading (non-medical prescribing) and SIFT fellow Oxford medical school. More recently she has also been teaching community matrons physical assessment skills.

Jill Davies, MSc Health Care Practice, PGdip Health Care Education, BA (Hons) Public Health Nursing, RN, RHV
Jill is Secretary of the local CPHVA branch with an interest in health visiting policy and practice. She is presently studying for a doctorate. The focus of this study is health visiting and prescribing. Although she works primarily as a lecturer, she still works in practice as a health visitor and nurse prescriber.

Sue Dundon, RGN, DN Cert, BA (Hons) Community Health Studies, CPT
Sue has worked as a District Nursing Sister for over twenty years. She became a Supplementary and Extended Prescriber in 2003 in Reading. She has always had an interest in Palliative Care and particularly in relation to patients with a non-cancer diagnosis. She now works as a Community Matron for Erewash PCT in Derbyshire.

Sue Garratt
Sue is employed as Lead Nurse Practitioner within a small team, which involves clinical input over several inner-city GP practices. A strategic focus contributes to the further development of Nurse Practitioners and Primary Care Nurses as community specialists within a PCT in Derby.

She is passionate about the difference nurses can make to the overall patient experience and providing patients with excellent care is her first and foremost aim in any intervention. She lives with her husband and two cats and enjoys reading, going out socially to nice pubs or eating lovely food, and travelling – especially within the Greek islands.

Anita Glenn, BSc (Hons) Nursing, PG Cert in Management Studies, Teacher Practitioner Cert, RGN, RMN, Community Mental Health Nursing Cert

Anita is Primary Care Manager Down/Lisburn HSS Trust and has been a nurse in a variety of settings for 36 years. She was seconded to the Nursing and Midwifery Group DHSSPSNI as Project Development Officer for Nurse Prescribing from 2001 to 2004 to take forward extended nurse prescribing in NI. She is married with two sons.

Matt Griffiths, RGN, BA (Hons), A&E Cert, FAETC, NISP
Matt is currently the Senior Charge Nurse in a Walk-in Centre and works for the Royal College of Nursing as a Joint Prescribing and Medicines Management Adviser.

He has been course leader for independent and supplementary nurse prescribing and supplementary pharmacists' prescribing courses. Matt is the Joint Secretary to the Nurse Prescribers' Formulary Sub-Committee (which advises UK Health Ministers on formulary inclusions); he is a founder member and helped to set up the MIMS for Nurses Editorial Board; and he is a member of the editorial boards of the *Journal of Community Nursing and Independent Nurse*. He was the Founding and Joint Editor of *Supplementary Prescribing* in *Practice*, and Founding Editor of www.prescriber-support.co.uk

He has published several papers on prescribing and co-edited a book with Dr Molly Courtenay. His political involvement in pushing for expansion of Non-Medical Prescribing means that he has submitted evidence to The House of Lords and Commons – Select committees, and was called as a witness to the Commons Health Select Committee. Matt has taken part in multiple focus groups and committees advising both agencies and ministers on aspects surrounding prescribing and medicines management.

Fiona Irvine
Fiona is Senior Lecturer in Nursing Research at the University of Wales, Bangor. She has a background in district nursing, health promotion and health education and worked as a district nurse and a Macmillan nurse before moving into nurse education, where her primary academic interest was community nursing. Fiona's work has now taken a research focus and her current research and writing relates to community nursing and to language and cultural awareness in health and social care.

Carol Kirkham MEd, Dip Ed, Cert Ed, HV Cert, NDN Cert, RGN
Carol is Lecturer in Nursing. She is special lead for all non-medical prescribing modules. Since 1990, she has been responsible for all practice nurse education at certificate, diploma and degree level including the Practice Nurse Pathway BSc (Hons) Health Studies, Specialist Practice award (since 1994). She is an external examiner/ moderator for the University of Glamorgan (prescribing courses).

Ruth Lonsdale, MSc Clinical Nursing, BSc (Hons) Community
    Nursing in the home, District Nursing, SRN, ONC
Ruth has worked in primary care since 1991. She worked as a practice nurse for some years and after qualifying through South Bank University then worked as a District Nurse. She then went on to work in a Walk-in Centre in Liverpool. In these roles, whilst working independently, there have always been wider team aspects to be considered especially in relation to prescribing. Ruth finds undertaking prescribing consultations both challenging and rewarding. Her knowledge of the types of conditions patients present with as well as that of drug therapies has broadened. Following her MSc, Ruth now works as a Nurse Practitioner in Elderly Rehabilitation, which enables her to continue to use consultation skills and prescribing within her professional practice.

Carolyn Mason, RGN, BA, PhD, RHV, RNT
Carolyn is Head of Professional Development in the Royal College of Nursing in Northern Ireland. She has a wide range of experience in community nursing, teaching and research.

Carolyn's main clinical experience is in health visiting and paediatrics. She has a degree and PhD in Social Anthropology, and has published many articles and contributed chapters on issues such as inequalities, primary care and research. She has recently worked for five years as a Nursing Officer in the NI Department of Health, Social Services and Public Safety, where she was responsible for the implementation of independent and supplementary nurse prescribing across Northern Ireland.

As Head of Professional Development, Carolyn leads the conference, library and information, and educational services for members of the RCN in Northern Ireland.

Ruth Oliver-Williams, MSc Evidence-Based Healthcare (Oxford), BSc (Nursing) Australia, RGN

After completing her 'hospital-based' training in 1990, Ruth commenced a career in Paediatric Oncology and Bone Marrow Transplant at the Welsh regional centre in Cardiff. In 1995, Ruth and her husband began a working adventure in outback Western Australia providing medical services to many diverse populations. Since returning to the UK in 2000, she has gained significant experience in a myriad of senior posts culminating in the Head of Nursing for Surgical Services in Slough. In December 2004 she successfully completed her Master's degree through Kellogg College Oxford, describing the experience as life changing. In January, Ruth, husband and Golden Retriever relocated to the Scottish Borders where she is the managing director of Evidence-Based Solutions Ltd, a health care consultancy.

Jenny Prior

Jenny commenced nurse training in 1981 at Nottingham, before moving to Scotland in 1985 and working in health care of the elderly in Edinburgh. She then undertook midwifery training and continued to work as a midwife in Glasgow where she has very fond memories of the old "Rottenrow". In 1992 she moved further north to the Orkney Isles and spent several happy years as a dual post community midwifery and nursing sister.

Jenny has been a midwife teacher at the University of Nottingham since 1997. She is Module Leader for biological and applied reproductive biological science. In addition to biology she lectures in pharmacology, HIV and AIDS and complications of childbirth.

The NMC requires midwife teachers to spend 20 per cent of time in clinical practice, which Jenny undertakes particularly in the community environment.

Penny Robinson

Qualifying from the London Hospital, Whitechapel in the 1960s, Pen Robinson has worked as a physiotherapist for four decades. After working for several years as both a clinical physiotherapist and a manager in the NHS, primarily in the long-term sector, Pen joined the Chartered Society of Physiotherapy in 1982 as the professional assistant to the Secretary, at that time the only employed PT within the CSP. In 1988 in recognition of the need to have an employed professional voice within the Society, the Professional Affairs department was formed. Pen led this department developing and building the professional profile of physiotherapy until her retirement in 2005. With an increasing number of professional staff, the CSP explored a number of areas of development for the profession to improve patient care including prescribing.

She now works part time for Capio Pinehill Hospital in Hitchin.

Jenny Rosalie

Currently Academic Dean for Nursing and Midwifery at The Academy Swindon. After qualifying as an RGN she went on to Study Midwifery. Much of her career has focused on Public Health and in particular Child Health, qualifying as a Specialist Practictioner in School Health in 2000 after undertaking a Master's Degree in Primary Care.

Following a Post Graduate Diploma in Education in Health and Social Care and qualifying as Practice Lecturer and educator, she now specialises in Education.

She is married with two children.

Ishbel Rutherford

Ishbel is Lecturer and Programme Leader for community health nursing at Queen Margaret University College, and has been involved in nurse prescribing since the introduction of initial prescribing for district nurses and health visitors in Scotland. She was a member of the Extended Nurse Prescribing Education Subgroup, for National Board for Nursing, Midwifery and Health Visiting, Scotland. Her other areas of interest are the use of portfolio development for learning and assessment and developing roles within community nursing.

Simon Sherring, RGN, RMN, BSc (Hons)

Simon works for South London and Maudsley NHS Trust, and is the Team Leader of an Assertive Outreach Team in Lewisham. He has worked in community mental healthcare for ten years.

Anne Sherry

Anne was trained at Glasgow Royal Infirmary 1977, after which she worked as a staff nurse and then a sister at the Royal Samaritan Hospital for Women in Glasgow.

Following this, she undertook midwifery training at Bellshill Maternity, and a degree in Community Specialist Nursing (GPN) in 2000, at Caldeonian University. Since becoming a practice nurse in 1987, she has undertaken the usual plethora of diploma level training in long-term conditions, and became a part-time coordinator of the nurse prescribing course at the QMUC two years ago after completing the leadership programme.

Her main interests are long-term conditions management and prescribing.

Millie Smith, MSc, Cert Ed, DNT, QN, RGN

Millie is now retired but was formerly Principal Lecturer at the University of Wolverhampton. Her responsibilities included subject leader for primary care, she was also postgraduate and undergraduate award leader for community specialist practice and nurse prescribing.

Sandy Tinson RGN, DipHV, DN cert, T Cert (Manchester), BSc, MSc

Sandy is a qualified district nurse and health visitor. She worked as a health visitor in both Oxfordshire and Buckinghamshire for several years before undertaking her teaching qualification and working as Lecturer at the University of Reading until 1998. She then returned to the NHS, initially as a professional development nurse and more latterly Director of Nursing. She was appointed to Reading PCT in 2001 as Director of Clinical Development, with a responsibility which included nursing, clinical governance, risk management, research, workforce planning and development.

Sandy's previous publications and research interests have focussed on health needs assessment, health promotion and clinical development. In her current role as Director of Quality, Standards and Workforce she is keen to ensure that the healthcare workforce has the necessary skills, knowledge and leadership to address the challenges within the new NHS.

Sue Topper

Sue Topper has had over 30 years' experience in primary care initially as a health visitor and then as a practice nurse. Following a move into higher education she was the course leader for the Extended and Supplementary Prescribing course for Nurses, Midwives and Health Visitors at the School of Health and Social Care at the University of Reading. Since this book was published she has returned to working for a local PCT.

List of abbreviations

AHPs	Allied Health Professionals
BHS	British Hypertension Society
BMA	British Medical Association
BTS	British Thoracic Society
CAS	Computer Assisted Software
CATS	Credit Accumulation Transfer Scheme
CCN	Community Children's Nurse
CD	Controlled Drugs
CM	Community Matron
CMP	Clinical Management Plan
COPD	Chronic Obstructive Pulmonary Disease
CPD	Continuing Professional Development
CSP	Chartered Society of Physiotherapists
CT	Computerised Tomography
DMP	Designated Medical Practitioner
DN	District Nurse
ESP	Extended Scope of Practice
GMS	General Medical Services
GSF	Gold Standards Framework
GSL	General Sales List
HEI	Higher Educational Institution
HPC	Health Professions Council
HV	Health Visitor
IP	Independent Prescribing
LCP	Liverpool Care Pathway
LDP	Local Delivery Plan
LTC	Long-Term Conditions
MIU	Minor Injuries Unit
NES	NHS Education for Scotland
nGMS	New General Medical Services contract
NICE	National Institute for Clinical Excellence

NMC	Nursing and Midwifery Council
NP	Nurse Practitioner
NPEF	Nurse Prescribers' Extended Formulary
NPF	Nurse Prescribers' Formulary for community practitioners
OOH	Out Of Hours Service
OSCE	Objective Structured Clinical Examination
PACT	Prescription Analysis and Cost
PAM	Professions Allied to Medicine
PCT	Primary Care Trusts
PGD	Patient Group Direction
PN	Practice Nurse
POM	Prescription-Only Medicines
PPC	Preferred Place of Care
PSD	Patient Specific Direction
QOF	Quality and Outcomes Framework
RPSGB	Royal Pharmaceutical Society of Great Britain
SHA	Strategic Health Authority
SI	Statutory Instruments
SN	School Nurse
SP	Supplementary Prescribing
TAS	Telephone Advice Software
WDD	Workforce Development Directorate
WHO	World Health Organisation
WIC	Walk-In Centre

Glossary of terms

Term	Definition
Acute NHS trusts	Hospitals that provide all secondary care services including accident and emergency facilities.
Administration of medicines	Administering a medication or medications to an individual patient.
Allied Health Professionals	Health care professionals other than doctors or nurses. Examples are physiotherapists, podiatrists, speech and language therapists, radiographers and so on.
Anticipatory prescribing	Providing a prescription for a patient in respect of symptoms that are likely to occur or become worse, often used in palliative care as part of schemes such as Liverpool Care Pathway.
BNF for children	Formulary containing information on prescribing for children.
British Hypertension Society	The British Hypertension Society provides a medical and scientific research forum to enable sharing of cutting-edge research in order to understand the origin of high blood pressure and improve its treatment.
British Medical Association	Regulatory organisation for doctors to ensure safe practice.
British Thoracic Society	Its core functions are descibed as: the relief of sickness of people with respiratory and associated disorders by the promotion of the highest standards of clinical care and the undertaking of research into the causes, prevention and treatment of respiratory and associated disorders, and disseminating the results of such research.
Case management	Case management is where a named coordinator, for example, a Community Matron, actively manages and joins up care by offering, amongst others, continuity of care, coordination and a personalised care plan for vulnerable people most at risk.
Cellulitis	Cellulitis is an infection of the skin and underlying tissues that can affect any area of the body.
Chartered Society of Physiotherapists	Regulatory body for physiotherapists.

Term	Definition
Chiropodist	Footcare Practitioner. State-registered chiropodists are those with a state-recognised qualification.
Chronic obstructive pulmonary disease	Chronic long-term and incurable condition of the pulmonary system causing reduced air exchange and poor oxygen perfusion.
Clinical governance	A framework through which NHS organisations are accountable for continuously improving the quality of their services and safeguarding high standards of care by creating an environment which encourages excellence in clinical care.
Clinical management plan	Written or electronic prescribing plans for individual named patients for management of specific conditions. They are agreed by an independent prescriber (doctor or dentist), supplementary prescriber and the patient to whom they apply. A Clinical Management Plan must be in place in order for supplementary prescribing to happen.
Community Children's Nurse	A Registered Children's Nurse who is also a qualified Community Specialist Practitioner.
Community matron	A nurse with advanced practice skills who is responsible for case management of patients with complex long-term conditions. Often patients have more than three long-term conditions and are at high risk of unplanned hospitalisation.
Co-morbidities	More than one long-term condition that may impact on other conditions.
Computer assisted software	Computerised algorithms to aid clinical decision-making.
Computerised tomography	CT scan (computerised tomography) also known as CAT scan (computed axial tomography) is a specialised x-ray test. It can give quite clear pictures of the inside of your body.
Concordance	Achieving an agreement with the patient through negotiation in order to gain a positive health benefit.
Continuing professional development	Activities undertaken by professionals to update knowledge and develop new skills and learning.
Controlled drugs	Prescription drugs subject to the Misuse of Drugs Regulations 2001, referred to as CD.
Co-terminus records	Patient records available at different locations.
Debridement	Debridement is the process of removing non-living tissue from pressure ulcers, burns, and other wounds.
Dependent prescribing	Prescribing as a supplementary prescriber under the auspices of a CMP agreed with a dependent prescriber and a patient.
Designated Medical Practitioner	A doctor who acts as a supervisor for a non-medical practitioner undergoing training.

District Nurse	A nurse with a specialist practitioner qualification who works in the community with patients who are mainly housebound.
EMIS	One of the computer systems available to general practitioners and other health care staff working in primary care. The systems are password protected and there are various levels of access in order to protect confidentiality.
Encoporesis	The repeated passing of stools into places other than the toilet – well past the time of normal toilet training.
Enuresis	Incontinence of urine at night.
Extended scope of practice	Extending the skills base of a practitioner through additional training.
First contact care	Providing the initial consultation when a patient presents for a consultation.
Fraser Guidelines	Criteria outlined by Lord Fraser in 1985 in the House of Lords' ruling in the case of Victoria Gillick versus West Norfolk and Wisbech Health Authority and the Department of Health and Social Security. They provide guidance for the assessment of the competency of minors in England to make health care decisions independently of parent or guardian.
General medical services	The GMS contract has evolved in partnership between the NHS Confederation and the General Practioners Committee (GPC) of the British Medical Association (BMA). It creates greater flexibility for GPs and represents an unprecedented level of investment in primary care.
General Sales List	Medicines that can be sold in pharmacies or supermarkets that are licensed for general sales to the public.
Gillick competency	See *Fraser Guidelines*.
Gold Standards Framework	The GSF improves the supportive palliative care of people towards the end of their life, and is used by primary health care teams to optimise the care provided for people living in the community, so that most care is delivered at home or to people attending GP surgeries.
Health Professions Council	Regulatory body for Allied Health Professionals.
Health Visitor	A qualified nurse working as part of the primary care team with a Community Specialist practitioner award.
Higher educational institution	Educational establishment that offers education across the spectrum ranging from undergraduate to postgraduate academic awards.
Independent prescribing	The prescribing of medicines by a health care professional autonomously. The prescriber is able to assess, diagnose and prescribe treatment for conditions. Independent prescribers are doctors, dentists, specially trained nurses and pharmacists. In relation to supplementary prescribing the independent prescriber is always a doctor or a dentist.

Term	Definition
Kaiser triangle	The 'pyramid of care' developed by US health provider Kaiser Permanente, which identifies the population of patients with long-term conditions into three distinct groups based on their degree of need.
Liverpool Care Pathway	The Liverpool Care Pathway for the Dying Patient was developed from hospice care for people in hospital and other settings. The LCP promotes good communication with patients and family, anticipatory planning including emotional, spiritual and psychological needs, symptom control and care after death.
Local delivery plan	Local delivery plans build upon capacity planning to develop local patterns for the capacity increases needed in the areas of workforce, physical facilities, and information management and technology.
Long-term conditions	Illnesses which lasts longer than a year, usually degenerative, causing limitations to one's physical, mental and/or social well-being.
Medical Supervisor	See *Designated Medical Supervisor*.
Minor injuries unit	A unit or clinic that may be nurse-led or operate within a Walk-in Centre or a hospital's Accident and Emergency Department. Patients are able to 'self' present with minor injuries and are assessed, diagnosed and treated or referred for specialist treatment.
Mode 1	A qualification obtained by a community nurse enabling them to prescribe from a limited formulary.
Mode 2	Similar to Mode 1 but the prescribing qualification is undertaken within the Specialist practitioner programme.
National Institute for Clinical Excellence	The institute is an independent organisation responsible for providing national guidance on promoting good health and preventing and treating ill health.
New general medical services contract	Contract negotiated between the DOH and GPs to deliver services in primary care.
NHS intranet	IT system accessed by employees of the NHS.
NHS npfit	The National Programme for IT in the NHS.
NHS plan (England)	The Plan published by the DOH in 2000 setting a 10-year strategy for investment and reform in the NHS.
Non-medical prescribing	Prescribing by practitioners other than doctors and dentists.

Nurse practitioner	A title given to nurses usually with advanced nursing skills who are able to provide complementary services in both acute and primary care settings. The title is soon to be regulated by the Nursing and Midwifery Council.
Nurse prescribers' extended formulary	Formulary devised to list those drugs prescribable by nurses who held the extended nurse prescribers qualification.
Nurse prescribers' formulary for community practitioners	A formulary that can be found in the Appendices of both the British National Formulary and the Drug Tarriff. This lists the medicines and appliances that can be prescribed by specialist community practitioners. It is updated monthly in the Drug Tarriff.
Nurse triage	A nurse undertakes an initial assessment of a patient in order to prioritise appointments. Initially used in Accident and Emergency Departments and now used in primary care settings. In some instances the nurse will give appropriate advice and treatment without the necessity for the patient to see a doctor.
Nursing and Midwifery Council	Regulatory body for nurses, midwives and health visitors.
Objective structured clinical examination	Practical or simulated examination which is part of he assessment process for those wishing to qualify as independent prescribers. Also used for other purposes.
Off-licence medicines	Those medicines contained in the BNF which are being prescribed for conditions or patients outside their licensed use.
Optometrist	Optometrists diagnose vision problems and eye disease, prescribe eyeglasses and contact lenses, and prescribe drugs to treat eye disorders. They cannot perform surgery, but they often provide patients with pre- and postsurgical care.
Out of hours service	Medical services offered in the evenings, at weekends and during bank holidays.
Palliative care	Total care of patients whose care is not responsive to curative treatments.
Patient group direction	A written direction for the supply and administration of prescription-only medicines to certain patient groups.
Patient specific direction	A prescription generated for a specific patient.
Pharmacist	A qualified professional knowledgeable about the pharmacology, supply, and administration of medicines who operates across a range of acute and community settings.

(Continued)

Term	Definition
Pharmacy (P) medicines	Medicines that can be bought 'over the counter' under the supervision of a pharmacist.
Pharmacy contract	Contract with the Department of Health to supply medicines.
Physiotherapist	Physiotherapists identify and maximise movement potential through health promotion, preventive health care, treatment and rehabilitation.
Pilot study	A study usually carried out prior to a full research study in order to test the tools and analysis methods that are to be used. Studies may be altered in response to the results from a pilot study.
Podiatrist	Specialist footcare practitioner.
Practice-based commissioning	Enables GPs to commission care and other services that will directly benefit patients registered with a GP surgery.
Practice nurse	A registered nurse employed in a GP surgery.
Pre-eclampsia	High blood pressure occurring in a pregnant woman that was not present before pregnancy. Often accompanied by fluid retention and can be accompanied by protein in the urine.
Preferred place of care	This is intended to be a patient-held record that will follow the patient through their path of care into the variety of differing health and social care settings. Guidance reference sheets for both the patient and carer and staff are available explaining the use of the PPC.
Prescribing	Deciding on a treatment for a patient and signing a prescription for that treatment.
Prescription analysis and cost	Data collected centrally to indicate prescribing patterns nationally and locally.
Prescription-only medicines	Those medicines only available on prescription.
Primary care trusts	Local NHS organisation responsible for the provision of primary care and community-based health services, services provided by family doctors, dentists, pharmacists, optometrists and ophthalmic medical practitioners, together with district nurses and health visitors.
Primary legislation	In the UK primary legislation is an Act of Parliament.
Professions allied to medicine	See *Allied Health Professional*.
Psychopharma-cology	The study of the effects of any psychoactive drug that acts upon the mind by affecting brain chemistry.

Public health	Public health is the branch of medicine concerned with the prevention and control of disease and disability, and the promotion of physical and mental health of the population.
Puerperium	The period usually lasting 6 weeks, following childbirth when the uterus returns to normal size.
Quality and Outcomes Framework	The QOF is a system of standards, incentives and assessment relating mainly to the essential and additional services delivered by GPs in primary care.
Radiographer	A qualified professional who performs radiography services and may operate as a disgnostic or therapeutic clinician.
Repeat prescription	A prescription issued to repeat medication following an initial consultation and generation of a prescription.
Royal Pharmaceutical Society of Great Britain	Regulatory body for pharmacisits.
Safety netting	A means of ensuring that all differential diagnosis options have been considered when conducting a consultation.
School nurse	A qualified nurse, who may hold a specialist practitioner qualification who works with children and offers services to school-age children.
Secondary legislation	Delegated legislation (sometimes referred to as secondary legislation or subordinate legislation) is law made by ministers under powers given to them by parliamentary acts (primary legislation) in order to implement and administer the requirements of the acts.
Skill mix	Teams comprised of practitioners with various qualifications.
Standing orders	Local guidelines produced by some maternity services to supplement authorisation of medicines that practicing midwives may supply or administer. This term does not exist in medical legislation.
Statin	Drugs that inhibit an enzyme involved in cholesterol synthesis. Effective in lowering LDL.
Statutory Instruments	Statutory Instruments (SIs) are what is known as secondary or subordinate legislation. They normally consist of an order, regulations, rules or a scheme and are made under powers conferred by primary legislation (an enabling Act).
Strategic Health Authority	The regional authority responsible for the allocation of NHS funds to the delivery of services for as defined population.
Supplementary prescribing	Prescribing medication within the confines of a clinical management plan which has been set up between an independent prescriber, a supplementary prescriber and the patient.
Supply of medicines	Supplying the medication either by dispensing or by selling the product to the patient.
Telephone advice software	Flow chart or algorithm used to guide clinical decision-making during a telephone consultation.

(Continued)

Term	Definition
Surestart	Surestart programmes are designed around local communities and focus on what local parents want.
Titration of medicines	The process of gradually adjusting the dose of a medication until the desired effect is achieved.
Travellers	Gypsies and Irish Travellers are recognised ethnic groups for the purposes of the Race Relations Act (1976), identified as having a shared culture, language and beliefs.
Unlicensed medicines	Medicines that currently do not have a licence for use. For instance new medicines that may be used as part of drug trials.
V100 prescriber	Nurses qualified to prescribe from the community nurses formulary.
V200 prescriber	A nurse who has been trained as an extended prescriber but not as a supplementary prescriber.
V300 prescriber	A nurse who is qualified as both an independent and a supplementary prescriber.
Walk-in centre	Walk-in centres offer quick access to a range of NHS services including free consultations, minor treatments, health information and advice on self-treatment. They are based in convenient locations that allow the public easy access and have opening hours tailored to suit modern lifestyles, including early mornings, late evenings and weekends.
Workforce development directorate	The department that allocates funding for workforce developemnt within PCTs.
Workforce planning	Planning exercise undertaken by Trusts to determine the resouce requirements for the delivery of services.
World Health Organisation	The World Health Organisation is the United Nations agency for health. It is governed by 192 member states grouped into six regions: Africa, Americas, the South-East Asia, Europe, eastern Mediterranean and Western Pacific.

Introduction

Dawn Brookes and Anne Smith

The purpose of this book is to provide health care professionals with a text that gives the factual information about non-medical prescribing, its evolution since first being suggested in the Cumberlege Report[1] and also to provide insights into the ways it has enhanced the roles of practitioners.

The implementation of prescribing in each of the four countries within the United Kingdom has been included as there are differences in the legislation that must be taken into consideration. Most of the contributors are reflecting on their roles within the NHS in England, which may differ from the prescribing role of practitioners elsewhere. It is essential therefore that the practices described here are considered within their context. The differences have been articulated within the contributions from individuals who are employed in the relevant countries. For example, independent prescribing is not an option in Wales as yet, although this is set to change in the near future.

It is hoped that this book will be a useful tool to examine how prescribing works in practice and is viewed by a variety of professionals, those already prescribing and those considering it. Case studies and practical examples, along with exercises throughout, illuminate the dialogue to demonstrate the innovations and improvements in service delivery facilitated by this qualification. The book will be of benefit to a wide range of health care professionals throughout the United Kingdom from both secondary and primary care.

The tone implicit within the text is of pragmatic implementation linked to critical appraisal. The subject is very topical and yet many practitioners are unaware of the revolution that is taking place. The book will therefore provide additional insight into all aspects of prescribing from workforce planning to practical implementation. A range of Clinical Management Plan templates in relation to supplementary prescribing have been included in order to help guide practitioners to develop their roles in this area. These are not meant to be used as they are presented as all such plans need to be developed for individual patients, taking into account an individual's medical history, allergies, other medicines and so on. They do, however, present a guide, using evidence-based practice at the time of writing.

The prescribing agenda is firmly placed within the overall NHS Plan confirmed within the Chief Nursing Officer's (CNOs) 10 key roles for nurses. The exciting developments regarding prescribing for pharmacists and other allied health professionals have been incorporated taking into account their views.

This book brings a unique addition to those already published and includes medical, strategic management, nursing and allied health professional perspectives as well as the contribution of an individual patient who eloquently describes the benefits of improved access and choice provided by extended and supplementary prescribing. In addition, due to the fact that health care professionals who wish to prescribe are required to be able to take a medical history and some need to be able to diagnose conditions, a chapter has been included providing information on consultation skills. Case scenarios provide some information relating to certain conditions and these provide useful insights into diagnostic reasoning. The contributors have therefore been drawn from all areas of health care where there is an interest in the progress of non-medical prescribing.

Part I begins with the historical aspects and moves on to give a guide to the modes of training and programmes available to prepare prescribers. A general practitioners' account of where prescribing partnerships fit in with the medical profession follows. This part concludes with discussions around target setting and workforce planning, explaining how non-medical prescribing could play a larger part in other NHS initiatives.

Part II describes the nursing and midwifery perspectives. It is mandatory that they become supplementary as well as independent prescribers. These chapters include case scenarios which will help those who may be considering prescribing to understand how and where it might enhance their current roles. Additionally it will help students of prescribing in the practical application of their studies. On the whole, pharmacology has not been included in this book as there are a number of pharmacology books available to students. Useful information, relating to prescribing has been included along with exercises that will help the reader to develop a knowledge base in this area.

Part III comprises the developments for allied health professionals (AHPs). A pharmacist explains how supplementary prescribing works in practice, independent prescribing is now a part of the pharmacists prescribing remit following training and this is considered. Other AHPs who have recently been given the opportunity to train as supplementary prescribers explain where they feel it will fit in with current practice and how it might evolve.

Part IV gives a wider perspective. It includes the issues of change management when implementing prescribing into a large secondary care organisation. Nurse triage is discussed in some detail. The subject of PGDs versus non-medical prescribing is tackled with the reader being more enlightened about the ethical and legal implications regarding the widespread use of PGDs presently adopted. The patient's experience is included and finally the important issues in relation to competency and accountability as a prescriber are discussed.

This is not a pharmacology book and neither does it seek to emulate other books previously published. It is, as the title suggests, a practitioner's toolkit with the aim of helping health care professionals to examine all of the issues in relation to non-medical prescribing. It aims to help them apply prescribing to practice and consider consultation models, differential diagnosis, clinical reasoning and prescribing implications as well as providing a 'how to' in various parts of the book. It is hoped that by reading this book or dipping into it, health care professionals will be able to make a more informed choice about how prescribing might benefit their practice and more importantly how it might benefit patients/clients. As editors, this is the type of book we would wish to have if we were considering either training in or application of non-medical prescribing.

There are still many anomalies that confuse practitioners as they embark on this path and it is therefore important that they can access support mechanisms to overcome the difficulties they may encounter. This text offers various resources to this end. However, individuals must accept personal responsibility to investigate problems and disseminate knowledge to the community of prescribers so that this skill will be a useful addition to their toolkit. It is important to acknowledge that the views contained in this book may not always be those of the editors. Chapter authors come from a variety of backgrounds and express how this subject has worked, is working or may work in their area of practice.

Reference

1. DHSS. *Neighbourhood Nursing: A Focus for Care* (Cumberlege Report) (London: HMSO, 1986).

Part I

Implementation of independent and supplementary prescribing in the United Kingdom

Chapter 1

Implementation across the United Kingdom

Policy Background
Molly Courtenay and Matt Griffiths

Recommendations were first made in 1986 for nurses to take on the role of prescribing. The Cumberlege Report[1] examined the care given to clients in their homes by district nurses (DNs) and health visitors (HVs). It was identified that some very complicated procedures had arisen around prescribing in the community and that nurses were wasting time requesting prescriptions from general practitioners (GP) for items such as wound dressings and ointments. The report suggested that patient care could be improved and resources used more effectively if community nurses were able to prescribe as part of their everyday practice, from a limited list of items and simple agents agreed by the Department of Health and Social Security (DHSS).

Following the publication of this report, the recommendations for prescribing and its implications were examined. An advisory group was set up by the Department of Health (DH) to examine nurse prescribing, which resulted in the first Crown Report.[2] Dr June Crown was the Chair of this group. The following is taken from this Report:

> Nurses in the community take a central role in caring for patients in their homes. Nurses are not, however, able to write prescriptions for the products that are needed for patient care, even when the nurse is effectively taking professional responsibility for some aspects of the management of the patient. However experienced or highly skilled in their own areas of practice, nurses must ask a doctor to write a prescription. It is well known that in practice a doctor often rubber stamps a prescribing decision taken by a nurse. This can lead to a lack of clarity about professional responsibilities, and is demeaning to both nurses and

doctors. There is wide agreement that action is now needed to align prescribing powers with professional responsibility.[2]

The report made a number of recommendations involving the categories of items which nurses might prescribe, together with the circumstances under when they might be prescribed. It was recommended that:

> Suitably qualified nurses working in the community should be able, in clearly defined circumstances, to prescribe from a limited list of items and to adjust the timing and dosage of medicines within a set protocol.[2]

Several groups of patients were identified that would benefit from nurse prescribing. These patients included: patients with a catheter or a stoma, patients with post-operative wounds and homeless families not registered with a GP. The Report also suggested that a number of other benefits would occur as a result of nurses adopting the role of prescriber. As well as improved patient care, this included better use of both nurses' and patients' time and improved communication between team members, arising as a result of a clarification of professional responsibilities.[2]

During 1992, the primary legislation permitting nurses to prescribe a limited range of drugs was passed.[3] Secondary legislation with necessary amendments were made to this Act, which came into effect in 1994, and a list of products available to the nurse prescriber was published in the Nurse Prescribers' Formulary (NPF) for DNs & HVs. In 1994, eight demonstration sites were set up in England for nurse prescribing. By the spring of 2001, around 20,000 DNs and HVs were qualified prescribers, and training programmes for DNs and HVs included the necessary educational component qualifying them to prescribe.

At the time of writing, there are over 28,000 DNs and HVs qualified to prescribe from a list of appliances, dressings, pharmacy (P) medicines (those products sold under the supervision of a pharmacist), and general sales list (GSL) items (those that can be sold to the public without the supervision of a pharmacist), and thirteen prescription only medicines (POMs) included in the NPF. Following a Nursing and Midwifery circular (NMC) in October 2005 other first-level nurses have been able to train as V100 prescribers in order to prescribe from what has now become the *NPF for Community Practitioners*.[4] In practice this means that, provided that there is an NHS need, school nurses, children's community nurses, practice nurses and occupational health nurses can undertake such training.

Extending Prescribing

A second report by Crown, which reviewed the prescribing, supply and administration of medicines, was published in 1999.[5] This review recommended that prescribing authority should be extended to other groups of professionals with training and expertise in specialist areas. During 2001, support was given by the government for this extension.[6] Funding was made available for other nurses, as well as those currently qualified to prescribe, to undergo the necessary training to enable them to prescribe from an extended formulary.

This formulary included:

- a number of specified POMs, enabling nurses to prescribe for a number of conditions listed within four treatment areas that were, minor ailments, minor injuries, health promotion and palliative care;
- GSL items used to treat these conditions;
- P medicines used to treat these conditions.

Further Extensions

During 2003, proposals by the Medicines and Healthcare Products Regulatory Agency (MHRA)[7] to expand the Nurse Prescribers' Extended Formulary (NPEF) were accepted and the NPEF was extended to include a number of additional conditions and medicines. In 2003, legislation was passed by the Home Office (HO) allowing nurses to prescribe six controlled drugs (CDs). These included:

- diazepam, lorazepam, midazolam (schedule 4 drugs) for use in palliative care
- codeine phosphate, dihydrocodeine and co-phenotrope (schedule 5 drugs).

Following further amendments to the Home Office Misuse of Drugs regulations and changes to the Prescription Only Medicines Order, further CDs and additional indications for existing CDs were added on 6 January 2006 and the total list is now as follows:[8]

- diamorphine, morphine, diazepam, lorazepam, midazolam, oxycodone for use in palliative care
- buprenorphine or fentanyl for transdermal use in palliative care
- diamorphine or morphine for pain relief for suspected myocardial infarction, or for relief of acute or severe pain after trauma, including in either case post-operative pain relief
- chlordiazepoxide hydrochloride or diazepam for treatment of initial or acute withdrawal symptoms caused by the withdrawal of alcohol from persons habituated to it
- codeine phosphate, dihydrocodeine tartrate or co-phenotrope.

See Appendix 1 for routes of administration and indications.

Proposals to extend the NPEF to include medicines and conditions in emergency and first contact care were accepted in 2004.[9]

Current Situation

The prescribing powers of nurses have greatly increased since the introduction of the original NPF. By January 2006 there were around 6100 extended nurse prescribers. These prescribers were able to prescribe from a list of over 250 POMs (including CDs), GSL and P medicines for a range of over 100 medical conditions. Following the results of proposals set out in early 2005,[10,11] Nurse Independent Prescribers (formerly extended nurse prescribers) are now able to prescribe any licensed medicine with the exclusion of CDs (except those listed earlier in this chapter). The prescribing powers of pharmacists have similarly increased, these health professionals are now able to train as independent prescribers.[11] Following the Medicines and Human Use (Prescribing) Order of May 2006, along with associated medicines regulations, nurses who have completed appropriate courses are able to prescribe any licensed medicine for any condition that falls within their competence.* At the time of writing this has been implemented in England and has been accepted in Scotland. Other devolved Governments of

---

*Improving Access to Medicines: A Guide to Implementing Nurse and Pharmacist Independent Prescribing within the NHS in England. Gateway reference 6429 (April 2006).

Northern Ireland and Wales are likely to implement the new legislation as they see fit. Legislation to allow pharmacists to become independent prescribers includes all licensed medicines but at the time of writing excludes prescription of CDs.

Supplementary Prescribing

The introduction of a new form of prescribing for professions allied to medicine was suggested in 1999.[5] It was proposed that this form of prescribing initially called 'dependent prescribing' would take place after a diagnosis had been made by a doctor and a Clinical Management Plan (CMP) drawn up for the patient. The term 'dependent prescribing' has since been superseded by 'supplementary prescribing'.[12]

A close partnership between the doctor and the nurse, pharmacist or Allied Health Professionals (AHP) is essential for the successful implementation of supplementary prescribing. Access to the patient's medical records and to a prescribing budget are other necessary pre-requisites. There are no legal restrictions on the clinical conditions for which supplementary prescribers (SPs) are able to prescribe. They are able to prescribe any medicine including CDs (nurses and pharmacists, in England only at the time of writing) and unlicensed medicines.[†]

Supplementary prescribing provides an ideal mechanism for treating some long-term conditions, including mental health problems. Where a team approach to prescribing is clearly appropriate, a CMP provides an ideal framework for prescribing for all those involved with the patient. Supplementary prescribing also provides a method by which newly qualified prescribers are able to develop their confidence in areas in which they feel less confident to prescribe independently.

Training for supplementary prescribing was introduced in 2003 for nurses and pharmacists, and legislative changes enabling the extension of supplementary prescribing to some physiotherapists, radiographers, podiatrists and optometrists are now in place.[13]

At the time of writing, there are over 6000 qualified nurse supplementary prescribers and over 500 qualified pharmacist supplementary prescribers.

[†]England only.

Although the literature examining supplementary prescribing is largely anecdotal, a number of themes are emerging. It is evident that there has been some confusion amongst some GPs and hospital doctors surrounding roles and responsibilities within the independent/supplementary prescribing partnership. The purpose of patient group directions (PGDs), protocols and CMPs, patient diagnosis and patient review (with regard to CMPs) are areas in which a lack of understanding has been identified.[14] Furthermore, the implementation of supplementary prescribing has been found to be time-consuming[15] and agreeing CMPs with GPs has been a big hindrance. Difficulties have also been experienced explaining the nature of supplementary prescribing to patients.[14] On a more positive note, people have confidence in the nurse having prescribed the best medicine for them, and say they would be willing to take it.[16] Further benefits reported include more effective use of nursing skills and the management of more complex cases by doctors[17] and a reduction in drug errors.[15]

The Benefits of Independent Prescribing

A small number of studies to date have been carried out to evaluate independent prescribing by nurses.[18] Some of the benefits reported by patients include accessibility and approachability of the nurse, the nurses' style of consultation, specialist expertise and information provision, and timely, convenient and continuous cares.[19–21] Benefits reported by nurses include more effective use of time, more convenient treatments and better information for patients, increased job satisfaction, status and autonomy, and the ability to deliver complete episodes of care.[19,20,22,23] Benefits of independent and supplementary nurse prescribing as viewed by doctors include improved professional relationships, a means of refreshing doctors' own knowledge, fewer interruptions to sign prescriptions and reduced workload.[24]

Influences on Independent Practice

A number of factors have been identified as influencing prescribing practice. These include inter-professional relationships, informal peer support gained through working in teams,[25–27] and awareness of the non-medical prescribers' role.[28]

Conclusion

Although the development of non-medical prescribing has been slow (prescribing by nurses first considered by the government during early 1980s), recent policy changes have meant that the role of the nurse, pharmacist and AHP with regard to prescribing has expanded dramatically over the last few years. The implementation of prescribing across the United Kingdom is discussed in the next part of this chapter with perspectives from Scotland, England, Wales and Northern Ireland.

References

1. DHSS. *Neighbourhood Nursing: A Focus for Care* (Cumberlege Report) (London: HMSO, 1986).

2. DH. *Report of the Advisory Group on Nurse Prescribing* (Crown Report) (London: DH, 1989).

3. DH. *Medicinal Products: Prescribing by Nurses Act* (London: DH, 1992).

4. NMC. V100 Nurse Prescribers. NMC Circular 30/2005SAT/lp (October 2005).

5. DH. *Review of Prescribing, Supply and Administration of Medicines* (Crown Report 2) (London: DH, 1999).

6. DH. *Patients to get Quicker Access to Medicines* (Press Release) (London: DH, 2001).

7. *MHRA* Consultation Document, MLX293, *NPEF* (2003).

8. Courtenay, M. Nurse prescribing update. *Journal of Community Nursing*, 2006, 20(2): 13–16.

9. MHRA. *Nurse Prescribers' Extended Formulary: Proposals to Expand the Range of POMs (MLX 320)* (2004).

10. MHRA. *Consultation on the Options for the Future of Independant Prescribing by Extended Formulary Nurses (MLX 320)* (2005a).

11. MHRA. *Consultation on Proposals to Introduce Independent Prescribing by Pharmacists* (2005b).

12. DH. *Supplementary Prescribing* (London: DoH, 2002).

13. DH. *Supplementary Prescribing by Nurses, Pharmacists, Chiropodists/Podiatrists, Physiotherapists and Radiographers within the NHS in England: A Guide for Implementation* (London: DH, 2005).

14. Baird, A. Supplementary prescribing: One general practice's experience of implementation. *Nurse Prescribing*, 2004, 2(2): 72–75.

15. Kinley, J. Nurse prescribing in palliative care: Putting training into practice. *Nurse Prescribing*, 2004, 2(2): 60–64.

16. Berry, D., Courtenay, M. and Bersellini, E. Attitudes towards, and information needs in relation to supplementary nurse prescribing in the UK: An empirical study. *Journal of Clinical Nursing*, 2006, 15: 22–28.

17. Hennell, S., Wood, B. and Spark, E. Competency and the use of CMPs in rheumatology practice. *Nurse Prescribing*, 2004, 2(1): 26–30.

18. Latter, S. and Courtenay, M. Effectiveness of nurse prescribing: A review of the literature. *Journal of Clinical Nursing*, 2004, 13: 26–32.

19. Brooks, N., Otway, C., Rashid, C., Kilty, E. and Maggs, C. The patients' view: The benefits and limitations of nurse prescribing. *British Journal of Community Nursing*, 2002, 6(7): 342–348.

20. Luker, K.A., Austin, L., Hogg, C., Ferguson, B. and Smith, K. Nurse-patient relationships: The context of nurse prescribing. *Journal of Advanced Nursing*, 1998, 28(2): 235–242.

21. Luker, K., Austin, L., Ferguson, B. and Smith, K. Nurse prescribing: The views of nurses and other health care professionals. *British Journal of Community Health Nursing*, 1997, 2: 69–74.

22. Rodden, C. Nurse prescribing: Views on autonomy and independence. *British Journal of Community Nursing*, 2001, 6(7): 350–355.

23. Latter, S., Maben, J., Myall, M., Courtenay, M., Young, A. and Dunn, N. An evaluation of extended formulary independent nurse prescribing. Executive summary of final report (London: DoH, 2005).

24. Avery, A., Savelyich, B. and Wright, L. Doctors' views on supervising nurse prescribers. *Prescriber*, 2004, 5: 56–61.

25. Humphries, J.L. and Green, E. Nurse prescribers: Infrastructures required to support their role. *Nursing Standard*, 2000, 14(48): 35–39.

26. Otway, C. The development needs of nurse prescribers. *Nursing Standard*, 2002, 16(18): 33–38.

27. Hay, A., Bradley, E. and Nolan, P. Supplementary nurse prescribing. *Nursing Standard*, 2004, 18(41): 33–39.

28. Pleasance, G. and Brownsell, M. Improving communication between nurse prescribers and community pharmacists. *Nurse prescribing*, 2004, 2(4): 171–173.

Further reading

Courtenay, M. and Griffiths, M. (eds). *Independent and Supplementary Prescribing: An Essential Guide* (Cambridge: Cambridge University Press, 2004).

Courtenay, M. Nurse prescribing update. *Journal of Community Nursing*, 2004, 20(2): 13–16.

Useful websites

www.doh.gov.uk/cno
www.npc.co.uk
www.mhra.gov.uk

Implementation in Scotland
Ishbel Rutherford and Anne Sherry

Jack McConnell, First Minister of the Scottish Parliament, referred to Scotland as 'one of the most unhealthy countries in Europe'.[1] Life expectancy in Scotland is lower than for the rest of the United Kingdom, with Glasgow having the lowest life-expectancy in the United Kingdom.[2] In addition, the proportion of life years spent with long-term health problems is higher, particularly in areas of deprivation.[3]

The future delivery of health care is a matter of national priority, and in his foreword to the National Framework for Service Change in the NHS,[4] Professor David Kerr summarises the Scottish context saying:

> Given the extraordinary health pressures that we face from a rapidly ageing population, dwindling birth rate, imposed working time directives from Europe, changes in working patterns, evolving technology and an ever expanding health gap between rich and poor, it should be obvious to all that the status quo definitely cannot be an option.

This and other recent policy documents[5] point to the development of a team approach to health care in Scotland, of which non-medical prescribing is one important aspect.

Nurse prescribing for DNs and HVs was introduced in Scotland in 1996,[6] extended nurse prescribing began in 2002 and supplementary nurse prescribing in 2003. At the time of writing, there are seven institutions of higher education offering the Independent and

Supplementary Nurse Prescribing course. Course delivery varies from predominantly taught days to distance learning to suit individual need. The University of Stirling offers electronic distance learning to accommodate the needs of practitioners working in remote and rural locations. This has now become available to a national audience via Emap.

Pharmacist prescribing began at the Robert Gordon University in Aberdeen in October 2003, and currently this University and Strathclyde University are offering training for pharmacists. Around one-hundred and fifty pharmacists have completed the course, with approximately two-hundred students studying at the time of writing. Independent prescribing for pharmacists was announced by Health Minister Andy Kerr in November 2005 to be in place by the spring of 2006.[7]

Legislative change to facilitate supplementary prescribing by other professions (optometrists, radiographers, podiatrists and physiotherapists) has been approved, and indicative content set. As yet, however, no Scottish institution is offering training for these groups.

It is worth noting that supplementary prescribers in Scotland are not (at the time of writing) able to prescribe controlled drugs or unlicensed drugs unless they are part of a clinical trial which has a clinical trial certificate or exemption.[8]

Institutions and individuals are supported by NHS Education for Scotland (NES), which has produced an excellent website. This site provides up-to-date interactive learning materials, which underpin course content in areas such as influences on and psychology of prescribing, legal policy and ethical aspects. It also offers a wide variety of applied pharmacology scenarios and case studies. See end of this section for website.

Uniquely in Scotland, nurse prescribing programme leaders have formed a networking group which meets twice a year to review the educational issues of implementing nurse prescribing. Scottish policy has been more cautious than in England, where it was suggested the majority of nurses would be able to use either independent or supplementary prescribing by 2004.[9] Two million pounds of central funding was allocated to train 1500 extended and/or supplementary prescribing nurses.[10] The NES database indicated that by January 2005, fewer than 500 students had completed the extended (now known as 'independent') and supplementary nurse prescribing course. At the time of writing, approximately two-hundred students are actively studying.[11]

Evidently the uptake of training has been less than anticipated. Currently there is little evidence available to identify reasons for this, but the British literature highlights criticism and concerns on a variety of levels ranging from the conceptual[12-14] to policy content and implementation.[15-17] Anecdotally, it seems there were several emerging themes from nurse prescribers. These included the limitations of the NPEF which is no longer an issue. Others pointed to practical difficulties in implementing supplementary prescribing policy, based on unrealistic assumptions, for example, that diagnosis is undertaken by doctors, and that medical review annually for large numbers of patients with long-term conditions is unworkable. Whilst there is limited evidence that some forms of nurse prescribing have been received favourably by professionals and patients,[18-21] the Scottish perspective is as yet unknown. Emerging evidence that many nurses may be underutilising[22] or not using[22] their prescribing powers is a cause for concern, and this aspect requires exploration.

The need for Scottish research is clear, and to this end the Scottish Executive has appointed a team at Stirling University to undertake a wide-ranging review of nurse prescribing in Scotland. This study will look at the impact of nurse prescribing on nurse prescribers, doctors, patients and other relevant groups. In addition the team aims to assess the learning experience of nurse prescribing students across Scotland and develop a typology of different curricular approaches.

In the meantime, existing nurse prescribers need to be supported in their new roles. This need has already been anticipated by the NES, which have launched a template for continuing professional development (CPD) that can be used by individuals or CPD providers.[23] The extent to which it has been used by nurses or health authorities, and therefore its value, is unknown at present.

Pharmacist supplementary prescribers are beginning to emerge, soon to be followed by pharmacist independent prescribers. The impact of this type of prescribing and how it will work in practice is yet to be seen. So is the impact of supplementary prescribing by AHPs.

There seems little doubt that Scotland has made good progress with the implementation of non-medical prescribing, though for reasons as yet unclear, not as much as expected. The level of clinical practice support for prescribers is incompletely understood, and a clearer picture of the barriers to prescribing should be developed in order to produce the policy changes which will allow non-medical prescribing in Scotland to reach its full potential.

References

1. British Broadcasting Corporation (BBC). *Scots Smoking Ban Details Set Out.* http://news.bbc.co.uk/1/hi/scotland/3999975.stm, accessed 01.02.05.

2. Hanlon, P., Walsh, D., Buchanan, D., Redpath, A., Bain, M., Brewster, D., Chalmers, J., Muir, R., Smalls, M., Willis, J. and Wood, R. *Chasing the Scottish Effect* (Scotland: Public Health Institute for Scotland/Information and Statistics Division, 2001). http://www.phis.org.uk/pdf.pl?file=pdf/chasing%20scottish%20effect.pdf, accessed 28.01.05.

3. Clark, D., McKeon, A., Sutton, M. and Wood, R. *Healthy Life Expectancy in Scotland* (On behalf of the HLE Measurement in Scotland Steering Group, 2004).

4. SEHD. *A National Framework for Service Change in the NHS in Scotland* (Edinburgh: SEHD, 2005).

5. SEHD. *Partnership for Care: Scotland's Health White Paper* (Edinburgh: SEHD, 2003). http://www.scotland.gov.uk/library5/health/pfcs-00.asp, accessed 01.02.05.

6. SEHD. Statutory Instrument No.1504 (S.132). *The National Health Service (General Medical Services, Pharmaceutical Services and Charges for Drugs and Appliances) (Scotland) Amendment Regulations* (Edinburgh: SEHD, 1996).

7. Scottish Executive. *Nurses get Greater Prescribing Powers* (Press Release). www.Scotland.gov.uk/News/Release/2005/11/11104434, accessed 13.02.06.

8. Scottish Executive. *Framework for Developing Nursing Roles* (Edinburgh: SEHD, July 2005).

9. DH. *The NHS Plan: A Plan for Investment, A Plan for Reform* (London: Department of Health, 2000).

10. SEHD. *Extended Independent Nurse Prescribing within NHS Scotland: A Guide for Implementation* (Edinburgh: SEHD, 2002).

11. Waddington, C. Personal Communication. 27.01.05.

12. Barker, P. Prescribing: The great debate. *Nursing Standard*, 2002, 17(9): 23.

13. Horton, R. Nurse-prescribing in the UK: Right but also wrong. *Lancet*, 2002, 359: 1875–1876.

14. Skidmore, D. Will you walk a little faster…? In: Humphries, J. and Green, J. (eds) *Nurse Prescribing*, 2nd edition, Chapter 9, pp. 129–139. (Basingstoke: Palgrave Macmillan, 2002).

15. Pickersgill, F. Extending nurse prescribing. *Primary Health Care*, 2001, 11(4): 23.

16. Mazhindu, D. and Brownsell, M. Piecemeal policy may stop nurse prescribers fulfilling their potential. *British Journal of Community Nursing*, 2003, 8(6): 253–256.

17. Baird, A. Recent developments in prescribing. *Journal of Community Health*, 2004, 18(3): 4–6.

18. Luker, K., Austin, L., Hogg, C., Ferguson, B. and Smith, K. Patient's views of nurse prescribing. *Nursing Times*, 1997a, 93: 515–518.

19. Luker, K., Willock, J. and Ferguson, B. Nurses' and GPs' views of the nurse prescribers' formulary. *Nursing Standard*, 1997b (22): 1133–1138.

20. Brooks, N., Otway, C., Rashid, C., Kilty, L. and Maggs, C. Nurse prescribing: What do patients think? *Nursing Standard*, 2001, 15(17): 33–38.

21. While, A. and Biggs, K. Benefits and challenges of nurse prescribing. *Journal of Advanced Nursing*, 2004, 45(6): 559–567.

22. Timbs, O. What pharmacists prescribers can learn from those who have gone before. *Prescribing and Medicines Management*, 2003, 5: 5.

23. National Health Service Education for Scotland (NES). *A Template for Continuing Professional Development in Prescribing* (Edinburgh: NES, 2003).

Further reading

Scottish Executive Health Department (SEHD). *Our National Health: A Plan for Action, a Plan for Change* (Edinburgh: SEHD, 2005).

Scottish Executive. *Framework for Role Development in the Allied Health Professions* (Edinburgh: SEHD, July 2005).

Further reading cont'd

Scottish Executive. *Framework for Developing Nursing Roles* (Edinburgh: SEHD, July 2005).

Useful websites

NHS Education for Scotland   www.nes.scot.nhs.uk/nursing/prescribing/default.asp

Scottish Executive   www.scotland.gov.uk

Implementation in Northern Ireland
Carolyn Mason and Anita Glenn

Northern Ireland is about the size of Yorkshire and has a population of 1.7 million. Given this relatively small area, it made sense to introduce non-medical prescribing consistently across the region. Prescribing by nurses is probably the most significant development in nursing since the inception of the NHS, testing ideas about 'which professionals do what' and ways of working that have become embedded over time.

Introducing nurse prescribing has been both challenging and rewarding. The challenge was led from the top by the then CNO Judith Hill. In 2001 a Project Officer was appointed to the government Department of Health, Social Services and Public Safety (DHSSPS) to carry out the work, under the leadership of one of the four Nursing Officers. In Northern Ireland, Health, Social Services and the Fire and Ambulance Services are combined into one government department, the DHSSPS. Protected project officer time was key to the success of implementation. An important feature of nurse prescribing is its interrelatedness with other aspects of health and social care, for example prescribing by nurses in primary care has an effect on practice-based prescribing budgets, and there are important implications for pharmacists who are legally accountable for ensuring the authenticity of prescriptions. This meant that a huge variety of detailed process issues had to be confronted, and a wide range of key stakeholders persuaded to commit to the change.

To drive the project, a senior level, multiagency, multiprofessional Steering Group was established, which included user representation as well as management, education and information computer technology (ICT) input. Although there was initially some resistance from individuals within clinical areas such as general practice, pharmacy and microbiology, there was full support from the Chief Medical Officer. Those who supported the initiative saw the potential for better access for patients and more efficient service delivery. Those who were cautious tended to emphasise risks around indemnity, adverse incidents and records management. Given these legitimate concerns and the key priority of patient safety, advice and expertise were needed from across the spectrum of primary, secondary and tertiary care, as well as legal, civil service and technological help, and, at top level, ministerial backing. An Education Sub-Group and an Implementation Sub-Group were established to bring this forward.

The independent and supplementary prescribing course in Northern Ireland is comprehensive and demanding, and it has generally been the case that multiprofessional colleagues who were initially sceptical about nurses' education and competence have been impressed. The course is offered as a part-time programme at degree or postgraduate level, lasting one year and it contains four modules:[1]

▶ Professional issues and patient empowerment
▶ Pharmacotherapeutics
▶ Health assessment
▶ Specialised assessment and prescribing.

A proportion of the programme consists of e-learning and students undertake 15 days of supervised practice.[2] Prerequisites to entry, as in other parts of the United Kingdom include support from a medical mentor and access to a prescribing budget. Northern Ireland has two universities and nurse prescribing is the first course ever to be offered jointly by these. From the outset, and in contrast to some other parts of the United Kingdom, the curriculum included both extended and supplementary prescribing and all students undertake both elements. Those who undertake the course come from a range of clinical areas and specialisms, including:

▶ nurse practitioners
▶ mental health nurses
▶ nurse specialists
▶ practice nurses

- midwives and
- accident and emergency (A&E) nurses.

Challenges for implementation have been, and continue to be, many. A distinct feature of Northern Ireland is the uncertain political situation. The disbandment of the NI Assembly in 2002 created a delay in passing the necessary legislation and amendments to associated regulations for nurse prescribing. In spite of this, the project has continued successfully and systems are in place to sustain expansion and development. Each of the four area Health and Social Services Boards has a designated Nurse Prescribing Adviser post, the education programme is well established and a nurse prescribing information system, NINA (Northern Ireland Nurse Analysis), has been built to capture information on nurse prescribing in primary care at individual, trust, board and regional levels.

There are still many challenges for non-medical prescribing in Northern Ireland. First, amongst these is the need to create a prescribing budget for these prescribers in primary care. Secondly, there can be a time lag between England and Northern Ireland in passing legislation and amendments to regulations to enable the prescribing. One such example is that of controlled drugs legislation which has only just been passed at the time of writing.[3] Supplementary prescribers are not yet allowed to prescribe controlled drugs, unlicensed or 'off label' drugs in Northern Ireland.[2] It is therefore important that websites are designed to make it easy for nurses and others to know which rules apply to each country, at any given time. In common with the rest of the United Kingdom, the bit-by-bit expansion of the formulary did create difficulties for practising nurses in knowing exactly what could be prescribed at a given moment. Professional guidance documents still need to be updated regularly.

As prescribing by nurses grows, the way is being paved for developments in practice that, only a few years ago, would have been unthinkable. Pharmacy colleagues have started supplementary prescribing and in due course will be joined by the AHPs.

Collectively, this promises to change the face of health care. Extended and supplementary prescribing is opening up the routes for nurses to diagnose, care and treat, and is empowering them to tailor the management of medicines to the needs of patients in a way that is beginning to realise the full potential of the nursing as a profession.

References

1. Department of Health, Social services and Public Safety (DHSSPS). *Extending Independent Nurse Prescribing within the HPSS in Northern Ireland: A Guide for Implementation* (Belfast: DHSSPS, April 2004).

2. DHSSPS. *Supplementary Prescribing by Nurses and Pharmacists within the HPSS in Northern Ireland: A Guide for Implementation* (Belfast: DHSSPS, April 2004).

3. Statutory Rule. *The Misuse of Drugs (notification of and supply to addicts) (Amendment) Regulations (Northern Ireland)* (Crown Copyright, December 2005). www.opsi.gov.uk/sr/sr2005/20050564.htm, accessed 18.02.06.

Useful websites

Department of Health, Social Services & Public Safety
www.dhsspsni.gov.uk

Implementation in England
Molly Courtenay and Matt Griffiths

Recommendations were first made in 1986 for nurses to take on the role of prescribing.[1] Eight years later (although limited to DNs and HVs, nurses in eight demonstration sites throughout England began to independently prescribe. At the time of writing, there are approximately 28,000 DNs and HVs qualified to prescribe from a list of appliances, dressings, Pharmacy (P), GSL items and POMs included in the Nurse Prescribers' Formulary (NPF). Other community specialist practitioners are now eligible to train for this type of prescribing.

The available research exploring nurse prescribing by DNs and HVs is positive.[2] Patients indicate that they are as satisfied, and sometimes more satisfied, with a nurse prescribing as they are with their GP.[3] Nurses and doctors report that they are able to use their time more effectively and that treatments for patients are more conveniently provided.[4,5] Nurses also report that they are able to provide patients with better information about their treatment and that they experience increased job satisfaction, status and autonomy.[5,6]

During 2001, funding was made available for all nurses, who met the agreed criteria, to undergo the necessary training to enable them to prescribe from an extended formulary.[7] Training for extended prescribing by nurses began in spring 2002. In 2003, proposals to expand the NPEF were accepted and the NPEF was extended to include a number of additional conditions and medicines.[8] In 2003, legislation was passed by the Home Office (HO) allowing nurses to prescribe six CDs.[9] Further CDs, included in the proposals set out by the MHRA,[8] have recently been added following HO approval. Additional proposals to extend the NPEF to include medicines and conditions in emergency and first contact care[10] were accepted in 2004 and came into effect in May 2005.

The result of recent proposals[11] to extend the NPEF yet further have been accepted, as have proposals to extend independent prescribing to include pharmacists.[12] These changes came into force on May 1st 2006.

Following DH approval in 2002,[13] training for supplementary prescribing was introduced in 2003 for nurses and pharmacists, and legislative changes enabling the extension of supplementary prescribing to some AHPs, physiotherapists, podiatrists, radiographers and optometrists are now in place.[14]

The benefits reported following the implementation of supplementary prescribing include, improved interprofessional relationships and more effective use of the skills of the SP (enabling the management of more complex cases by doctors),[15] reduction in drug errors,[16] and standardisation of treatment across groups of patients.[17]

In England, at the time of writing, there are over 6000 independent/supplementary nurse prescribers and over 500 supplementary pharmacist prescribers.

References

1. DHSS. *Neighbourhood Nursing: A Focus for care* (Cumberlege Report) (London: HMSO, 1986).

2. Luker, K.A., Austin, L., Hogg, C., Ferguson, B. and Smith, K. Nurse-patient relationships: The context of nurse prescribing. *Journal of Advanced Nursing*, 1992, 28(2): 235–242.

3. Latter, S., Maben, J., Myall, M., Courtenay, M., Young, A. and Dunn, N. *An Evaluation of Extended Formulary Independent Nurse Prescribing: Executive Summary.* www.dh.gov.uk/publicationsandstatistics/pressreleases, accessed 29.06.05.

4. Brooks, N., Otway, C., Rashid, C., Kilty, E. and Maggs, C. The patients' view: The benefits and limitations of nurse prescribing. *British Journal of Community Nursing,* 2001, 6(7): 342–348.

5. Luker, K., Austin, L., Ferguson, B. and Smith, K. Nurse prescribing: The views of nurses and other health care professionals. *British Journal of Community Health Nursing,* 1997, 2: 69–74.

6. Rodden, C. Nurse prescribing: Views on autonomy and independence. *British Journal of Community Nursing,* 2001, 6(7): 350–355.

7. DH. *Patients to get Quicker Access to Medicines* (Press Release) (London: DH, 2001).

8. MHRA. Consultation Document, MLX293, NPEF (2001).

9. HO. 40/2003. *An amendment to the Misuse of Drugs Regulations 2001 – To Permit the Prescribing of CDs by Nurses in Restricted Circumstances, and the Supply of PGDs in Accordance with a PGD* (London: HO, 2003).

10. MHRA. *Nurse Prescribers' Extended Formulary: Proposals to Expand the Range of POMs* (MLX 320) (2004).

11. MHRA. Consultation Document, MLX 320, NPEF (2005a).

12. MHRA. *Consultation on Proposals to Introduce Independent Prescribing by Pharmacists* (2005b).

13. DH. *Supplementary Prescribing* (London: DH, 2002).

14. DH. *Supplementary Prescribing by Nurses, Pharmacists, Chiropodists/Podiatrists, Physiotherapists and Radiographers within the NHS in England: A Guide for Implementation* (London: DH, 2005).

15. Hennell, S.L., Wood, B. and Spark, E. Competency and the use of CMPs in rheumatology practice. *Nurse Prescribing,* 2004, 2(1): 26–30.

16. Kinley, J. Nurse prescribing in palliative care: Putting training into practice. *Nurse Prescribing,* 2004, 2(2): 60–64.

17. Baird, A. Supplementary prescribing: One general practice's experience of implementation. *Nurse Prescribing,* 2004, 2(2): 72–75.

Implementation in Wales
Fiona Irvine and Carol Kirkham

Historical Background

Following the Cumberledge Report of 1986[1], a review of community nursing in Wales in 1987 led to the production of 'Nursing in the Community – A Team Approach for Wales',[2] which recommended that 'legislative changes should be made to allow nurses to prescribe from a limited formulary agreed with the Medical profession' (p. 48). These recommendations finally came into force in Wales in January 2001 when the first cohort of community nurses (district nurses and health visitors) began prescribing.[3]

Supplementary Prescribing

Before the initiation of nurse prescribing in Wales, the concept of supplementary prescribing was already being considered and the second Crown Report[4] recommended that prescribing powers be extended to nursing groups other than community nurses with a district nursing or health visiting qualification and to other professionals, such as pharmacists and therapists. A distinction was made between independent prescribers, who would be responsible for the initial assessment of the patient and subsequently drawing up a treatment plan, and supplementary prescribers, who would be authorised to prescribe for patients whose condition had been previously diagnosed by an independent prescriber, within the parameters of an agreed treatment plan. In May 2001 the Department of Health (DH) announced that prescribing authority would be extended to allow practitioners to prescribe treatments for a wider range of medical conditions from an expanded formulary. By March 2003 they published the implementation guide for supplementary prescribing by pharmacists and nurses, and in England training for supplementary prescribers began in 2003. Whilst the training in Wales was the same as that in other parts of the United Kingdom, nurses were not allowed to independently prescribe from the NPEF.

Overview of Supplementary Prescribing Education Programme in Wales

With the support of the Welsh Assembly Government, the decision was taken to develop a single All Wales Curriculum for *supplementary prescribing*, for pharmacists and nurses employed in Wales. An underpinning theme of the curriculum is that nurses and pharmacists are taught together and assessed using the same criteria. Thus the taught programme meets the relevant standards set by the Nursing and Midwifery Council (NMC) and the Royal Pharmaceutical Society. The programme is designed to develop the critical analysis and personal reflection skills of the students and to prepare them for continuous professional development.

The curriculum is normally delivered over a six-month period and comprises of 90 hours (15 days) taught contact, 72 hours (12 days) learning in practice and 218 hours of directed study. The module attracts 20 credits at level HE3.

The programme is developed around four main themes, namely: communicating, consultation and decision-making, therapeutics and clinical governance. Communicating seeks to prepare students to enhance their ability to communicate effectively across professional boundaries and to work in partnership with key individuals to achieve concordance. Consultation and decision-making prepare students to undertake assessment and diagnosis and to generate treatment options within a clinical management plan. The theme of therapeutics addresses safe and effective prescribing using an appropriate management plan. It also considers patient monitoring and referral. Finally, clinical governance prepares students to work within a clinical governance framework in relation to supplementary prescribing.

A rigorous assessment strategy underpins the programme and consists of an Objective Structured Clinical Examination (OSCE) and a practice portfolio comprising of:

1. A needs analysis, action plan and diagnostic essay
2. A clinical log and reflective critical analysis of cases from practice
3. Three clinical management plans.

Progress to Date

In Wales, it was agreed that a maximum of two cohorts per year would undertake the training with a maximum of 30 students entering the programme at each one of five educational providers in Wales. The first cohort of nurses and pharmacists commenced training as supplementary prescribers in March 2004. They completed the programme in December 2005 and successful students were awarded a Certificate in Supplementary Prescribing. They register with the NMC (nurses) or the Royal Pharmaceutical Society (pharmacists) as Supplementary Prescribers, before beginning to prescribe. The second student cohort commenced the programme in January 2005.

The success of supplementary prescribing in Wales is yet to be established since the first cohort of successful students is just beginning to prescribe. However, it is anticipated that the extension of supplementary prescribing to a wider range of nurses and pharmacists is a major step in ensuring that patients receive comprehensive and seamless care from the most appropriate professional.

A recent announcement by Health Minister Dr Brian Gibbons gave a commitment to introduce independent prescribing by pharmacists and nurses in Wales. This progression is eagerly awaited.[5]

References

1. DHSS. *Neighbourhood Nursing: A Focus for Care* (Cumberledge Report) (London: HMSO, 1986).

2. Welsh Office. *Nursing in the Community: A Team Approach for Wales* (Edwards Report) (Cardiff: Welsh Office, 1987).

3. Green, J. *Development of the Nurse Prescribing Initiative.* In: Humphries, J. and Green, J. *Nurse Prescribing*, 2nd edition. (Basingstoke: Palgrave, 2002).

4. DH. *Review of Prescribing, Supply and Administration of Medicines* (Crown Report 11) (London: DH, 1999).

5. Welsh Assembly. *Independent Prescribing Coming to Wales.* Press Announcement (19 January 2006). www.Wales.gov.uk/Servlet/PressReleaseByDate/Servlet?area_code, accessed 29.01.06.

Chapter 2

Educational preparation for the prescribing role

Sue Topper

Introduction

This chapter will examine the educational preparation required for different types of non-medical prescribing programmes, the course content and assessment processes. National guidance for the selection of those who wish to extend their role and how this can be implemented will also be covered.

The situation in relation to prescribing has been complex. The history of this initiative has been documented in Chapter 1, however, it may be beneficial to outline the training methods by which different health professionals can become prescribers.

Different Types of Qualifying Courses

Nurses

Community Practitioner Nurse Prescribers (Formally District Nurse and Health Visitor Prescribers) V100

District nurse (DN), health visitor (HV) and practice nurses with a DN or HV qualification who have undertaken educational preparation fall into this category (Mode 1 prescribing). The training is now integrated into the Specialist Practitioner Community programme (Mode 2 prescribing) and is available to all nurses undertaking this training, including school nurses, community paediatric nurses and practice nurses. Stand-alone courses are no longer available; however, community specialist practitioners, through local arrangement, may attend the prescribing element of specialist practitioner programmes.

Having completed the programme practitioners can prescribe anything from the Nurse Prescribers' Formulary for Community

Practitioners (formerly the Nurse Prescribers' Formulary for District Nurses and Health Visitors – NPF).[1] These nurses assess, diagnose and prescribe treatment without recourse to a doctor and manage a whole episode of care independently. The qualification is recorded (annotated) on the NMC Register as V100 prescriber.

Exercise

Examine a copy of the British National Formulary (BNF) that includes the NPF and find this section in the Appendices. Look up the contents. Consider how much this formulary contributes to autonomous practice. List the prescription only medicines (POMs) that are available through the formulary along with their indications and side effects.

Extended Nurse Prescribers (V200)

An outline curriculum of the educational preparation for extended prescribing was produced by the English National Board (ENB) for Nursing and Midwifery in September 2001.[2] The Nursing and Midwifery Council (NMC) has developed standards for the approval of courses offered by Higher Education Institutions (HEIs) across the United Kingdom[3]. These new standards were developed to take into account the expansion of this type of prescribing to include that of the whole of the BNF.

Prior to the introduction of supplementary prescribing, nurses, midwives and health visitors who completed the extended prescribing courses were recorded on the register as V200 prescribers and this remains so unless they undertake the required extra training to become supplementary prescribers. This training is no longer available singularly.

Nurse Independent/Supplementary Prescribers (V300)

Nurses who were V200 prescribers and undergo extra study and assessment to undertake supplementary prescribing become both independent and supplementary prescribers (SP). See Chapter 3 for definition. The training is now combined and nurses must undertake the whole programme. On successful completion of the course the qualification is recorded on the NMC Register as a V300 prescriber.

Nurse Independent Prescribers (NIP) work as independent prescribers in that they assess, diagnose and prescribe treatment

autonomously and manage whole episodes of care. They origin-
ally prescribed from the NPEF, prescribing only for the conditions
listed. They are now able to prescribe from the whole BNF, with
the exception of CDs* and unlicensed drugs for conditions that fall
within their competence (see Chapter 19). At the time of writing,
nurses and pharmacists are the only health professionals, other
than doctors or dentists, who can independently prescribe.

Interprofessional Education

In HEIs across the United Kingdom, training for extended
prescribing is now combined with that for SP. Presently multiprofessional education is offered in England and Wales only.† The
Royal Pharmaceutical Society of Great Britain (RPSGB), responsible
for validating SP programmes for pharmacists has acknowledged
that much of the SP curriculum is common to both nurses and
pharmacists.[4] (See Chapter 12 for further details.)

Since October 2005, AHPs in England have also been trained for
supplementary prescribing alongside pharmacists and nurses. The
first courses to be validated were those in Trent. Optometrists have
chosen to train independently and do not currently join with the
other professional groups.

At the time of writing, health professionals who can train as
supplementary prescribers are nurses, pharmacists, physiotherapists, radiographers, chiropodists and optometrists.

Exercise

Find out whether there are any nurses in your area of work that are qual
ified prescribers. How often are they prescribing and what items are most
common?

Pharmacists

At the time of writing, pharmacists, having undertaken an education programme recognised by the RPSGB or the Pharmaceutical

---

*Some controlled drugs can be prescribed for certain indications. See www.
dh.gov.uk
†See NMC Position Statement. www.nmc.org.uk

Society of Northern Ireland (PSNI), are able to undertake training to become supplementary and independent prescribers. Previously they were able to qualify as SPs having undertaken the training.

Pharmacists who successfully complete the course may apply to the Registration Section of the RPSGB within six months of the date of the award and following a registration fee will be annotated on the RPSGB Register of Pharmaceutical Chemists as supplementary/independent prescribers. See Chapter 12 for further discussion.

AHPs

Changes to the Prescription Only Medicines Order and NHS regulations in 2005[5] have enabled supplementary prescribing responsibilities to be extended to other groups of AHPs,* following a period of training.

These are:

- chiropodists/podiatrists
- physiotherapists
- radiographers
- optometrists.

Chiropodists/Podiatrists

Following various amendments and changes in the law over the last thirty years, podiatrists and chiropodists have been able to obtain and administer local analgesics (LA) in the course of their professional practice. These approved podiatrists have LA rights identified on their registration certificate issued by the Health Professions Council (HPC). Some podiatrists may also hold a certificate of competence in the use of other specified medicines, and are able to obtain and supply these to patients in the course of their professional practice.[5]

Many podiatrists use PGDs to support their clinical work especially when involved in surgical practice or in the conservative

---

*Not yet available in Northern Ireland.

management of the high risk foot.[5] A PGD enables the practitioner to *supply and administer* the medication within a protocol for patients who meet a set criteria. This differs from a CMP which is patient specific and where the practice of *prescribing takes place*. See Chapter 18.

Members of the Society of Chiropodists and Podiatrists who are in possession of the above certificates are obliged to undertake periodic continuing professional development in both Local Anaesthesia and Pharmacology for Podiatrists, Access and Supply.[5] The first podiatrists to complete supplementary prescribing did so in February 2006. See Chapter 14 for more information.

Physiotherapists

Physiotherapists, as part of their pre-registration course, develop various skills in relation to a basic knowledge of pharmacology relating to a limited range of medicines. These may relate to medicines management or may be more applied to demonstrate the interrelationship between drug therapy and physiotherapy intervention.[6]

Other physiotherapists may have undertaken further study to enable them to use injection therapy to manage musculoskeletal injuries or have experiential knowledge of a range of medicines related to their area of expertise.[5] See Chapter 13 for further information.

Radiographers

Diagnostic Radiographers

During their pre-registration training diagnostic radiographers gain a thorough knowledge and understanding of the pharmacology of medicines commonly encountered within imaging settings with a particular emphasis on contrast agents, associated medicines and pharmaceuticals and the methods of the administration of medicines.[7]

Therapeutic Radiographers

During their pre-registration training these radiographers gain a thorough knowledge of the pharmacology of medicines commonly used for the relief of symptoms encountered within an oncology setting. These include cytotoxic drugs, hormonal agents, imaging contrast agents and radiopharmaceuticals. They will also have an understanding of their methods of administration. See Chapter 15 for further information.

Following successful completion of the course an AHP will be annotated as a supplementary prescriber on the HPC Register. See Chapter 15 for further information.

Exercise

Speak to a health professional, outside of your profession, who has completed the training as a supplementary prescriber. Discuss how this has enhanced their role. Make a list of conditions for which supplementary prescribing might be useful and spend time developing one patient specific CMP relevant to your clinical practice. Template available at: http://www.dh. gov.uk/PolicyAndGuidance/MedicinesPharmacyAndIndustry/Prescriptions/ NonmedicalPrescribing/SupplementaryPrescribing/Supplementary PrescribingArticle/fs/en?CONTENT_ID=4123030&chk=t3E8Fk

Optometrists

Optometrists are among the professionals covered by exemptions to the Medicines Act 1968. These exemptions allow them to sell or supply in an emergency the following:[8]

- GSL medicines
- P medicines
- POMs (not for parenteral use) which:

  1. are eye drops containing not more than 0.5 per cent chloramphenicol
  2. are eye ointments containing not more than 1 per cent chloramphenicol
  3. contain atropine sulphate, bethanecol chloride, carhachol, cyclopentolate hydrochloride, homatropine hydrobromide, naphazoline nitrate, physostigmine salicylate, physostigmine sulphate, pilocarpine hydrochloride, pilocarpine nitrate and tropicamide.

Optometrists are also among the AHPs who can train to be supplementary prescribers. They expect to be given independent prescribing rights soon after.[9]

Selection of Potential Prescribers

The Department of Health suggests that the selection of those wishing to undertake training as prescribers should be a matter for local decision but those selected *must* have the opportunity to prescribe in the post they will occupy once they have completed the training.[10]

Key principles that should be used to prioritise potential applicants are:[11]

- patient safety
- maximum benefit to patients and the NHS in terms of quicker and more efficient access to medicines for patients
- improved quality of care
- increased patient choice in accessing medicines
- better use of professionals' skills
- contribute to flexible working across the NHS.

Normally, close collaboration between the employer and the funding authority is crucially important to ensure that the right candidates are sent on prescribing training courses.[10]

In practice those needing to write a prescription in order to complete an episode of care for a patient should be considered.

Pharmacists and AHPs have specific knowledge relating to their specialisms and would be able to incorporate this into their practice by being non-medical prescribers. These issues are discussed in more detail in the relevant chapters.

Funding

In England central funding has been made available through Strategic Health Authorities (SHA), Workforce Development Directorates (WDDs) to meet the costs of training. It is for these organisations to decide how this funding is best used to ensure the required numbers of professionals are trained.

In Scotland potential candidates apply to their employing operating division and funding has been provided through the Scottish Executive Health Division (SEHD) and is reviewed annually. Funding in Wales comes from the Welsh Assembly. In Northern Ireland it comes direct from the DHSSPS.

Pharmacists and AHPs apply to their employing organisation or if self-employed, may need to be prepared to meet the costs of the course themselves. In England funding may be made available to the independent sector where there is likely to be benefit to NHS patients. For example pharmacists and nurses employed by a hospice.

Exercise

Consider the role extension that is made possible by becoming a prescriber. In what way is this acknowledged by management and colleagues? What are the incentives to take on this responsibility within your role?

Educational Preparation

The following is applicable across the United Kingdom. Northern Ireland (NI) is, at the time of writing, passing legislation allowing AHPs to become supplementary prescribers but it is envisaged that it will be the same as for the rest of the United Kingdom.

It is recommended that wherever possible, training for prescribing should be interprofessional. Where HEIs are offering courses for nurses it is hoped that these can be combined to include some joint teaching with pharmacists and other AHPs.

The requirements laid down by the NMC state that the course to qualify nurses to prescribe as extended and supplementary prescribers should be of at least 38 days duration. This should consist of 26 taught days and 12 days learning in practice with additional learning time in self-directed study.[3] HEIs in NI require 15 days clinical experience. The programme should be completed in 6 months and only in exceptional circumstances can this be extended to 12 months, although in NI the training is over an academic year.

The RPSGB and PSNI requirements for pharmacists supplementary prescribing training was that there should be at least 25 days face-to-face teaching and no less than 12 days of learning in practice.[12] As pharmacists are now independent prescribers, courses are being amended to include appropriate training and assessment and the length of training has not been confirmed at the time of writing. This is the reverse of the situation that arose in nursing, when practitioners converted from the V200 course, it is likely that 2 extra days of training will be necessary to enable them to prescribe independently.

The DH and the HPC suggest that the programme for AHPs should be at least 26 days with 12 days learning in practice over a period of no more than 12 months.[5]

The training is usually undertaken over a period of three to six months, in some cases a day per week and others in blocks of learning a week at a time.

The combined course for nurses in England attracts between 30 and 45 credit accumulation and transfer points (CATs) at Level 3/6 (degree), or Level 4/7 (Masters). This varies according to accreditation processes within the HEIs. Other countries such as Northern Ireland are able to award a greater number of credits and some offer up to 60 credits.[4] For AHPs it is likely to attract 30 CATs at level 3/6 and for pharmacists 30 credits at level 4/7.[12]

The assessment criteria is by:

▶ examination (minimum 80 per cent pass mark to be achieved)
▶ portfolio/learning log
▶ satisfactory completion of practice experience
▶ Objective Structured Clinical Examination (OSCE) in a simulated learning environment or examination of practice in a relevant setting or a video consultation in a live practice setting
▶ numeracy assessment (100 per cent pass mark).

Even if the above is achieved the health professional must be referred if they fail to answer a question correctly that may result in direct harm to a patient/client.[3]

Where appropriate the production of a CMP to be used in practice is examined as part of the assessment process. The issues for service providers in relation to the training of prescribers are considerable. Students are very often senior practitioners in their field, and releasing them for the period of study has serious staffing implications. Table 2.1 shows the requirements that need to be met by those applying for training in prescribing.

Distance Learning

Nurses

A number of HEIs offer programmes which have a distance learning element. This information can be obtained by contacting specific HEIs for information about course delivery. Due to the

Table 2.1 Requirements for those wishing to become prescribers

Requirements	Nurses and midwives	Pharmacists	Allied health professionals
Registration	Current Registration on Parts 1, 2 or 3 NMC Register	Current Registration with RPSGB/PSNI	Current Registration with HPC in one of the relevant Allied Health Professions
Professional practice	Should have the required knowledge of the area in which they wish to prescribe. One year working in the relevant practice area preceding application. Occupy a post in which they will be expected to prescribe	Pharmacists should ensure that their knowledge, skills and performance are current and relevant to their field of practice	Should be practising in an environment where there is an identified need for the individual to regularly use supplementary prescribing
Support from employer	Written agreement from their employing organisation that they will be supported when undertaking the programme. Employer is responsible for ensuring nurses are able to undertake a history, assessment and diagnosis if they are not undertaking a module preparing them in diagnosis and physical assessment alongside the prescribing module[3]	Obtain the agreement of their sponsoring authority that a supplementary prescribing partnership will meet service need, for example by enabling progress towards access targets or local health strategies	Should be able to demonstrate support from their employer/sponsor including confirmation that the entrant will have appropriate supervised practice in the clinical area in which they are expected to prescribe
Approved Medical Practitioner	Written confirmation of the support from a designated medical practitioner who is able to commit time (12–15 days)	Access to a medical supervisor who has experience in the relevant field of practice, training and experience in	Access to a medical supervisor who has experience in the relevant field of practice, training and experience in

	and to assess the learner's progress in practice	the supervision, support and assessment of trainees and who agrees to provide learning opportunities and supervise, support and assess the student during the clinical placement	the supervision, support and assessment of trainees and who agrees to provide learning opportunities and supervise, support and assess the student during the clinical placement
Post registration experience	At least 3 years post registration experience	At least 2 years experience as a pharmacist, following pre-registration year after graduation. Not the case in Northern Ireland as entry can be immediately after qualifying	At least 3 years relevant post-qualification experience
Educational criteria	Ability to study at level 3/6. In Northern Ireland candidates require 60 credits at level 2/5	Ability to study at a minimum of QAA level 3/6	Ability to study at a minimum of level 3/6

geography of the country of Scotland, HEIs there were among the first to offer distance learning programmes. See Chapter 1.

Emap in conjunction with the University of Stirling[13] offers an e-learning programme for nurses, which is designed to enable them to study in a more flexible way. The amount of study required is the same but the amount of face-to-face contact is reduced from 26 days to a minimum of 10, the rest of the time being self-directed study. The amount of supervised practice is the same (12 days) and a medical supervisor is required to ensure the learning outcomes are achieved in practice. Programmes must clearly demonstrate how the learning outcomes will be met. For students who prefer self-directed learning such courses offer a greater degree of flexibility than traditionally taught courses. Department of Health requirements for distance learning programmes (England) is for 8 face-to-face taught days (excluding assessment) and 10 days protected learning time.[14]

Pharmacists

Materials from the Centre for Pharmacy Postgraduate Education (CPPE) are available to support pharmacists undertaking the prescribing programme.[12] This does not reduce the amount of face-to-face contact required to complete the programme, but the materials are a useful supplement. The three modules are presented as self-contained units drawing together and relating to the knowledge, skills and attitudes needed to support the acquisition of the learning outcomes.[12] Exercises, practice scenarios and case studies are used to support the achievement of the learning outcomes.

For further details visit http://www.cppe.man.ac.uk

AHPs

In England, AHPs began training from October 2005 with the first courses to be validated in Trent and the first professionals joining the course at the University of Derby. At the time of writing, there are no distance learning courses for this professional group.

Course Content

Areas of study to be covered in the curriculum include:[3]

- consultation, decision-making and therapy including referral
- influences on and psychology of prescribing including concordance
- prescribing in a team context
- legal, policy and ethical issues
- clinical pharmacology including the effects of co-morbidity
- evidence-based practice and clinical governance in relation to non-medical prescribing
- professional accountability and responsibility
- prescribing in a public health context.

Continuing Professional Development (CPD)

All the professional bodies (NMC, RPSGB and HPC) highlight the importance of CPD for prescribers. The National Prescribing Centre (NPC) has produced a range of CD ROMs for health professionals to support their continuing professional development (CPD), which can be obtained from http://www.npc.co.uk. Further information can be found in Chapter 19.

Exercise

Reflect on the attitudes of the other professionals with whom you work. Are they aware of the possibilities that are available once you are trained as a non-medical prescriber. Are the medical practitioners in favour of the concept and willing to act as mentors? Perform a SWOT (Strengths, Weaknesses, Opportunities and Threats) analysis to persuade a manager of the advantages.

Conclusion

Challenges for HEIs include the wide range of practitioners wishing to access the courses. The profile of prescribing is rising within the health care professions. Some doctors are very supportive and are happy to provide supervision for prescribing students, others are less so and some are opposed to the concept.

Some health care professionals still prefer to work under the auspices of PGDs but the UK Governments have made it clear that it is preferable and safer for medicines to be prescribed rather than be supplied under PGDs.[10] The supply and administration of medicines under PGDs should be reserved for those situations where this offers an advantage for patient care and where it is consistent with appropriate professional relationships and accountability (see Chapter 19).

Recent years have seen a change in those nurses and pharmacists wishing to undertake the preparatory training. Participants are less likely to be from primary care as consultant and specialist nurses, along with hospital pharmacists, are realising the opportunities that prescribing can bring. Since the widening of the scope of prescribing in practice through opening up the BNF to nurses and independent prescribing for pharmacists this trend is likely to continue for some time to come.

References

1. Department of Health. *Nurse Prescribers' Formulary.* www.dh.nhs.uk, accessed 12/07/05.

2. English National Board for Nursing, Midwifery & Health Visiting. *Education Policy Letter 2001/01/TL* (London: ENB, 2001).

3. Nursing and Midwifery Council. *Standards of Proficiency for Nurse and Midwife Prescribers* (London: NMC, 2006). www.nmc.org.uk, accessed 02/05/06.

4. Courtenay, M. and Griffiths, M.*Independent and Supplementary Prescribing: An Essential Guide* (London: Greenwich Medical Media, 2004).

5. National Prescribing Centre/Department of Health. *Outline Curriculum for Training Programmes to Prepare Allied Health Professional Supplementary Prescribers* (London: DH, 2004).

6. Chartered Society of Physiotherapy. *The Curriculum Framework for Qualifying Programmes in Physiotherapy* (London: CSP, 2002).

7. College of Radiographers. *Framework for Professional Development* (London: SOR, 2003). www.sor.org, accessed 12/07/05.

8. Buckley, R., Lawrenson, J. and Hennelly, M. 'Recent developments in drug legislation for optometrists.' *Optometry Today*, January (2005) 40–46.

9. Steele, C. and Johnson, P. 'Extended clinical roles and PGDs: Putting theory into practice. *Optometry Today*, February (2005) 30–32.

10. Department of Health. *Supplementary Prescribing by Nurses, Pharmacists, Chiropodists/Podiatrists, Physiotherapists and Radiographers within the NHS in England: A Guide for Implementation* (London: DH, May 2005).

11. Brookes, D. 'Selecting and developing extended nurse prescribers'. *Nurse Prescribing* 2: 5 (2004) 212–216.

12. Royal Pharmaceutical Society of Great Britain. Supplementary Prescribing. http://www.rpsgb.org.uk/memebers/medicines/supplpresc.htm, accessed 13/07/05.

13. Emap. Nurse Prescribing Programme. www.archive.hsj.co.uk/OpenLearning/nurse.htm

14. DH. *Improving Patients' Access to Medicines: A Guide to Implementing Nurse and Pharmacist Independent Prescribing within the NHS in England* (London: DH, 2006). www.dh.nhs.uk, accessed 03/05/06.

Useful websites

Health Professions Council	www.hpc-uk.org
College of Pharmacy Practice	www.collpharm.org.uk
National Electronic Library for Health	www.nelm.nhs.uk
Royal Pharmaceutical Society of Great Britain	www.rpsgb.org.uk/members
Nursing and Midwifery Council	www.nmc.org.uk

Chapter 3

Prescribing partnerships: a GP perspective

Helen Crawley

Introduction

This chapter will discuss areas involving prescribing partnerships from a GP's perspective. Whilst primary care is the author's area of expertise some reference will be made to areas in secondary care where non-medical prescribing may benefit service delivery.

Doctors and dentists are no longer the only health care professionals who can prescribe. Nurses and pharmacists can now prescribe independently and they, along with other professionals, can train to become supplementary prescribers. Hospitals are beginning to benefit from prescribing partnerships which have become commonplace in primary care. General practice is an ideal setting for non-medical prescribing. Practice nurses and nurse practitioners are increasingly acting as the first point of patient contact, dealing with both 'on the day' appointment requests and the management of long-term conditions. Judicious use of non-medical prescribing allows nurses to take professional responsibility for the prescriptions they sign and to spend more time with patients. General practice can also benefit from pharmacists undertaking the prescribing role and carrying out medication reviews within the surgery. Prescribing partnerships with community pharmacists are also possible but tend to be more problematic.[1]

Prescribing partnerships with nurses, pharmacists and AHPs in secondary care settings are likely to improve the patient's journey through the health care system and provide greater job satisfaction to the professionals involved. Podiatrists will be able to treat patients with conditions where they have expertise and the same applies to physiotherapists and radiographers. Some of these partnerships could be extended into primary care where there are AHPs working closely with GPs or in community hospital settings.

Exercise

Consider the other professional groups who you are in regular contact with. Examine a scenario of a patient journey in which several professionals are involved and determine who may be the most appropriate person to prescribe for them.

New General Medical Services Contract

The new General Medical Services contract (nGMS)[2] includes a points system outlined in the Quality and Outcomes Framework (QOF). The contract was agreed between the BMA's General Medical Practitioners' Committee and the NHS Confederation on behalf of all four UK countries. This framework enables GPs to be remunerated for achieving standards in four domains:

1. clinical standards
2. organisational standards
3. additional services standards
4. patient experience.

The clinical standards domain includes a range of long-term conditions, which could potentially be managed by non-medical prescribers. Organisational standards include medicines management such as reviews of repeat prescriptions, which non-medical prescibers could undertake as part of their management of long-term conditions. The access patients have to primary care health professionals can gain points for GP practices in the organisational and patient experience domains. Appropriate use of non-medical prescribing can improve patient access to the primary care team. The additional services domain includes areas such as contraceptive services, immunisation and smoking cessation advice.

For GPs, there are considerable opportunities to benefit financially under nGMS from non-medical prescribing.[3,4] For patients, there is the potential for improved access and seamless care, with the most appropriate health care professional seeing them and providing a prescription, and for nurses, pharmacists and AHPs there is the chance to develop professionally and take on new roles.

Exercise

The nGMS Contract has influenced the way primary care services are delivered. How might non-medical prescribing benefit patients accessing out of hours services?

Nurse Prescribing in General Practice

The principles in this section, whilst focussing on primary care, are equally valid in secondary care practice.

The extended formulary for nurses initially concentrated on minor ailments, minor injuries, health promotion and palliative care.[5] Health promotion included preconception counselling, contraception, emergency contraception, smoking and vaccinations. The list of diseases and medicines covered by the extended formulary continued to expand from 2002[6] and now includes all medicines in the BNF for nurses in England and Scotland to prescribe from as long as the disease area is within their competence.[7,8] Northern Ireland and Wales are expected to have the same provisions in the near future. Where CDs and unlicensed medicines are used nurses and pharmacists will still need to enter into supplementary prescribing partnerships.

Practice nurses have traditionally undertaken health promotion activities and the treatment of patients with minor injuries not presenting at accident and emergency departments. In addition, many nurses are now working effectively as the first point of contact for undiagnosed patients presenting in primary care.[9] The management of minor illnesses by practice nurses acting in this domain is a cornerstone of the drive towards 'advanced access', with all patients being able to see a primary care professional within 24 hours.[10,11] See Chapters 5 and 17 for more information about access.

Prescribing allows nurses to complete an episode of care including the consultation and treatment where appropriate without recourse to a doctor. Nurses are thus able to work autonomously in areas where they have already developed professional knowledge and experience. They are acting as independent prescribers, taking full responsibility for diagnosis and appropriate prescribing.

Before independent nurse prescribing, nurses always had to get the 'rubber stamp' of a doctor's signature in order to issue a prescription. Although the doctor signing the prescription took legal responsibility for it, in practice there was often little discussion around the prescribing decision. Nurses felt, quite correctly, that they were professionally covered by the medical practitioner. Doctors often signed prescriptions without really questioning the full implications of their actions. There was a potential risk of patient harm as neither the doctor nor the nurse felt fully accountable for the issuing of a prescription. The potential for drug errors may be reduced when appropriately trained nurses sign their own prescriptions.[12]

There is a danger that nurses might feel less welcome to interrupt GP colleagues for advice about patients who appear to have conditions they should be able to prescribe for, even when the nurses are not entirely certain about the diagnosis or management. Hopefully, a reduction in the frequency of interruptions for routine signatures will ensure that GPs are willing to provide excellent support to their nursing colleagues on the rarer occasions when their opinion is sought. As ever, good interpersonal relationships and professional respect are the keys to successful patient care within the primary care team.

As well as dealing with health promotion, minor illnesses and minor injuries, most practice nurses and more recently community matrons and district nurses are involved in the monitoring and management of patients with long-term conditions. Nurses are able to effectively manage long-term problems such as Parkinson's disease, diabetes mellitus, chronic obstructive pulmonary disease, bronchiectasis,[13] coronary heart disease and heart failure to name but a few.[14] Some examples of monitoring potential long-term conditions are listed below.

- Mental health including depression.[15] The importance of monitoring patients before issuing prescriptions with the potential for overdose means that patients with mental health problems are suitable for supervision by appropriately trained nurses.
- Newly diagnosed or uncontrolled conditions such as diabetes, asthma, coronary heart disease, heart failure, hypertension,[16] chronic obstructive pulmonary disease, hypothyroidism, polymyalgia rheumatica[17] and so on, where frequent monitoring

and dose changes or changes in medication are likely to be necessary.

▶ Conditions which require frequent monitoring of blood tests for safe prescribing with possible alterations in dosage such as warfarin anticoagulation,[18] lithium[15] and disease-modifying antirheumatic drugs.[17]

▶ Patients with a previous history of coronary heart disease or cerebrovascular events in whom appropriate prescribing can reduce the risks of recurrence. Examples would include reviewing patients with a history of coronary heart disease who are not currently taking beta blockers.

Exercise

Using these examples map your involvement in the management of any of these groups of patients. Is there, or would there be, a significant difference in your management if you can/could prescribe within the consultation. As you read on determine the benefits of supplementary prescribing in comparison with independent prescribing

Pharmacist Prescribing

Pharmacists are already involved in primary care long-term conditions management.[18–20] Conditions where extensive physical examination is not necessary, such as cardiovascular risk factor control, warfarin monitoring or the treatment of hypertension, are most likely to be suitable for pharmacists, especially those working in community pharmacies.

Supplementary Prescribing

By using a CMP,[21–23] supplementary prescribers across the United Kingdom are able to prescribe for any condition from the whole of the BNF; in England this includes CDs and unlicensed medicines prescribed as part of clinical trials. Nurses and pharmacists no longer need to formulate CMPs in many cases although some may still prefer to do so. Partnerships with GPs and hospital consultants remain paramount in order to provide safe prescribing relationships and lack of repetition and alteration by doctors who still have ultimate responsibility for medical management of patients.

Supplementary prescribing is 'a voluntary partnership between an independent prescriber (a doctor or dentist) and a supplementary prescriber to implement an agreed patient-specific Clinical Management Plan with the patient's agreement'[21] (paragraph 6). The independent presciber is responsible for the 'initial clinical assessment of the patient, the formulation of the diagnosis' and for 'carrying out a review of the patient's progress at appropriate intervals, depending upon the nature and stability their condition'[21] (paragraph 19). The independent and supplementary prescriber should 'ideally, jointly carry out the formal clinical review at the agreed time – normally within 12 months . . . (Periods longer than 12 months between joint clinical reviews or reviews by the independent prescriber may *occasionally* be acceptable in the CMP where the patient's condition has been shown to be stable . . .)'[21] (paragraph 15).

Although supplementary prescribing has limitations, it does allow non-medical prescribers to complete consultations for long-term conditions management, including providing appropriate prescriptions.

Conditions Suitable for Supplementary Prescribing

Supplementary prescribing allows medication dosage to be altered or new medicines to be introduced within a CMP. The conditions which most lend themselves to supplementary prescribing are those in which frequent reviews are necessary.[24] It would be appropriate to set up CMPs for patients with conditions that may require dose titration or where treatments can be anticipated. Such treatments can then be managed by supplementary prescribers. Examples can be found in Appendix 2 of this book.

The supplementary prescriber must only work within the limits of their own clinical competence.[11] The conditions which individual prescribers manage will depend upon their own professional expertise. Generally speaking, health care professionals will simply continue to review the same patients as before, but will be able to sign prescriptions. Indeed, the transition to supplementary prescribing is likely to be most straightforward when the supplementary prescriber is already seeing the patients they plan to prescribe for.[19]

Supplementary prescribing is also suitable for health promotion prescribing and might include unlicensed prescriptions such as tricycling combined oral contraceptive pills. GPs may be particularly keen to involve non-medical prescribers in areas for which they gain points under nGMS.[2]

Communication in Prescribing Partnerships

Communication is essential for safe prescribing. The non-medical prescriber must share, consult and keep up to date the same common patient record. For supplementary prescribing the independent and supplementary prescriber must both have access to any guidelines or protocols referred to in the CMP.[21] All those treating the patient should have access to the CMP.[24]

For nurses and pharmacists working in a surgery, contemporaneous access to patient records presents no problems. Many GPs already have a close working relationship with a pharmacist, for example in those practices with a pharmacy on the same site. For these pharmacists, access to records should not be problematic and prescribing partnerships should be relatively easy to set up.[25]

In secondary care where notes are available to all parties there should be no problems in relation to supplementary prescribing partnerships. AHPs running clinics should have access to the same records as the hospital consultant and communication can be shared through these notes.

CMPs used in supplementary prescribing can either be handwritten or typed, for example, as an 'off the shelf' proforma following national guidelines which are then customised for individual patients. These CMPs can be signed and scanned in[24] or set up on the computer with a code added to confirm agreement of the prescribers.[18] There is also potential for electronically generated CMPs. If the supplementary prescriber has any doubts as to whether continued prescribing under the CMP is appropriate, they should be able to contact the independent prescriber. A decision can be made about discontinuation or continuation of the CMP, or the writing of a new one. In practice, if the independent prescriber who signed the CMP is not available, the supplementary prescriber may contact another independent prescriber and start a new CMP after jointly reviewing the patient.

Community pharmacists find it more problematic to share patient records. Connection to the NHS intranet has solved some of these problems for some pharmacists who are able to communicate changes in medication to the relevant GP.[18] The proposed information technology system for the NHS 'npfit' patient record should improve record keeping and sharing further.[26]

Potential Problems and Solutions

How Many Doctors and Supplementary Prescribers Should Sign the CMP?

Supplementary prescribing allows for more than one independent prescriber and supplementary prescriber to agree to a CMP[21] (paragraphs 16, 22, 53). There are some advantages to having only one independent prescriber responsible for each one. If more than one signs it, there may be difficulties ascribing professional liability if problems arise. A close relationship between a trained supplementary prescriber and one independent prescriber may enhance the supervision of the supplementary prescriber, but can leave other doctors within the GP practice or hospital team confused about the role of the supplementary prescriber.[24] On the other hand, if only one independent prescriber signs the CMP, it will come to an end if that person leaves the practice or the hospital team.[21] In addition, if the independent prescriber who agreed the CMP is not available when a supplementary prescriber has a problem, a new one will have to be agreed between a different doctor (who must review the patient), the patient and the supplementary prescriber.

In some primary care practices, only one GP has signed each CMP, either because it relates to their patient or because the GP has a special interest or responsibility for the clinical area the CMP covers. In other practices, more than one GP may sign a CMP.

How Should Clinical Reviews be Set up?

Before a CMP is initiated, the independent prescriber should make a diagnosis.[21] It is important not to miss reviews by the independent prescriber as the CMP becomes invalid once this date is passed.

Some practices use paper-based systems to track review dates.[24] Other practices have devised systems where one doctor is responsible for each disease area, and all patients in that clinical area have their CMPs reviewed in the same month each year.

What About Patients with More Than One Disease?

Many patients suitable for non-medical prescribing have co-morbidities. In the past, issuing repeat prescriptions for multiple pathologies involved simply printing out the prescription for all repeats requested and getting it signed by the doctor. If the non-medical prescriber feels unable to prescribe all a patient's repeat medicines, they could issue and sign one prescription for the items listed in the CMP and produce a second prescription on a different prescription, listing the rest of the items requested. They will then have to obtain the doctor's signature. This will tend to discourage non-medical prescribing as no time is saved. If the nurse or pharmacist is happy and competent to sign for all the medication a patient regularly uses, they may do so. They may not, however, be happy to make any dose or medication changes if the condition is one with which they are not as familiar and would refer back to the GP. The same issues may arise in secondary care as a nurse admitting a patient to a ward may not feel competent to enter all of the patient's usual medication onto a drug chart and may only be entering a small proportion thereby non-medical prescribing becomes less advantageous. Arguments may arise about the competence of a junior house officer to prescribe all a patient's usual medication, too, but as this has been standard practice for years it is less likely to attract undue attention.

Involving the Patient in Decision-making and Consent

Patients must consent to supplementary prescribing.[21] Many patients have not objected because they had assumed that nurses were always able to prescribe. Bellingham[18] and Baird[24] reported that consent for supplementary prescribing has been readily given. Obtaining consent from those with a poor grasp of english had been challenging at times. Baird[24] suggests an advice slip is given to patients, and gives an example of the slip she devised which could overcome the language barrier if translated.

Exercise

The previous section has highlighted some important issues relating to the development and management of CMPs. What do you think is best practice? Consider your accountability and legal responsibilities as a prescriber in relation to the discussion.

Administrative Problems

Prescription Production – Repeat and Acute

Between consultations with the supplementary prescriber, the practice may be issuing repeat prescriptions. It may be easier for interim repeat prescriptions to be issued under a doctor's name and signed by a GP, in the same way that other repeat medication requests are issued. The prescription must otherwise be dealt with separately from other repeat requests. GPs can sign each others' prescriptions but should not sign those of a supplementary prescriber. The problems of issuing repeat prescriptions are compounded if patients request several items at once, only some of which can be signed by the supplementary prescriber. Some practices may find it easier to remove supplementary prescribing from the procedure for repeat prescription issuing.

Pharmacists Not Issuing Items

It had been reported[24] that some pharmacists were unaware of the extent of supplementary prescribing and did not issue prescriptions for items requested. Pharmacists working near a practice with a supplementary prescriber did not pose a problem as they were personally aware of the arrangements. As non-medical prescribing becomes more widespread this should become much less of a problem.

Prescription Pads and Budgets

Delays of several months before registration of prescribing qualifications and the issue of prescription pads have been reported[12] although this situation is improving.

For nurses and pharmacists employed by practices, prescribing will be from the surgery budget. DNs and HVs also prescribe from this budget. For community pharmacists, obtaining a budget from the local NHS provider can be much more problematic.[18] AHPs will be prescribing from their employing organisations' budgets as their partnerships are likely to come from within these areas.

Medical Practitioner Concerns

Many medical colleagues see prescribing by other health professionals as a logical step. It acknowledges the abilities of these professionals and clarifies issues of professional accountability. Other doctors see non-medical prescribing as dangerous and unwelcome.

Other potential problems with increased prescribing by nurses have been identified by Hay and Bradley.[26] These include reduced opportunities for the training of junior doctors to manage and prescribe for simpler cases. In the author's experience the nursing team is so well developed in some practices that GP registrars have little exposure to 'simple' cases such as patients with urinary tract infections or for hypertension reviews as they are managed almost exclusively by nurses. Other concerns included the suspicion that prescribing was a cynical attempt to overcome a lack of doctors and the possibility of duplication of roles within a team.

In practices with a good skill mix which have embraced non-medical prescribing, the role of the GP is likely to change. They may deal with the more complex cases, oversee other members of the primary care team, review patients on CMPs[4] and undertake clinical audit and protocols. Some GPs have responded to the change in complexity of the cases they see by increasing the length of their consultations. GPs may also offer second opinions on patients for whom AHPs are the first point of contact, or may have more problematic cases triaged to them by other doctors or nurses.

Most of general practice is currently run by self-employed principals who see themselves as managing any innovations in their practices, such as the introduction of prescribing by their non-medical employees and colleagues. For some nurses, access to a prescription pad is seen as part of the process of empowering their profession, allowing them to initiate improvements in primary care services and become involved in business and management roles, rather than waiting subserviently to be delegated tasks by doctors.[4,23] However, other nurses seem reluctant to move from providing to planning patient care.[26] In the future, doctors may feel that the professional hierarchy (which they are used to being at the top of) is uncomfortably challenged as nurses, pharmacists and other AHPs take more of a lead in providing health care services.

Exercise

There has been a great deal of comment about the extension of prescribing in the media and particularly in the professional journals. Search the literature for some of the reporting and analyse the comments according to the publication in which they have been printed.

Where community pharmacists set up clinics separate from GP surgeries, GPs may feel particularly threatened. Enhanced services such as warfarin monitoring could quite easily be undertaken in community pharmacies, with payment for these services moving from GP surgeries to pharmacies.

Conclusion

There are many advantages to non-medical prescribing. The writing of CMPs can improve patient care. Writing a CMP forces supplementary and independent prescribers to agree on how an individual patient or particular long-term condition should be managed. Nurses have described how this has clarified patient care and brought some unity between individual GPs and the nursing team. CMPs tend to be evidence based, so writing them is an opportunity to review current management options providing best practice.

For nurses, pharmacists and AHPs there is the opportunity to develop professionally. By working in a team together, professional accountability is clearer when the person who generates a prescription also signs it. And for doctors there is the opportunity to work alongside skilled professionals, in a team, and to focus on longer consultations with those patients who cannot be managed as effectively by other members of the primary care team.

The benefits for patients include earlier access to improved care. In some areas, pharmacists are reviewing patients when they come to collect repeat prescriptions. Pharmacists have been able to offer open access to patients who are poorly controlled or fail to attend their GP for conditions such as asthma or hypertension.[18] With nurse run-clinics, nurses can prescribe rather than waiting for prescriptions to be signed. Prompt treatments can be provided by non-medical prescribers in the acute sector thus reducing waiting and patient suffering which can only be beneficial to patient satisfaction and outcomes.

References

1. Andalo, D. 'Pharmacists in St Helens take on new services in advance of contract deal'. *Prescribing and Medicines Management*, July: 1–4. www.pjonline.com (accessed 31/3/05).

2. NHS Confederation, British Medical Association. *The New GMS Contract: Investing in General Practice* (London: The NHS Confederation, 2003).

3. Crawley, H. 'How nurse prescribers will help practices gain quality points'. *Pulse*, March 15 (2004) 42–43.

4. Rashid, C. 'The new GMS contract: What does it mean for supplementary prescribing?' *Nurse Prescribing*, 2: 1 (2004) 6–8.

5. Department of Health. *Extension on Independent Nurse Prescribing* (2002a) http://www.doh.gov.uk/nurseprescribing/pomlist.htm (accessed 31/3/02).

6. British Medical Association/Royal Pharmaceutical Society of Gt. Britain. *British National Formulary*. No. 49 (London: BMA/RPSGB, March 2005).

7. Department of Health. *Nurse & Pharmacist Prescribing Powers Extended* (Press Release). www.dh.gov.uk/PublicationsAndStatistics/PressReleases/ PressReleasesNotices/ (accessed 4/1/06).

8. Scottish Executive. *Nurses get Greater Prescribing Powers* (News Release). www.scotland.gov.uk/News/Releases/2005/11/11104434 (accessed 4/1/06).

9. Horrocks, S., Anderson, E. and Salisbury, C. 'Systematic review of whether nurse practitioners working in primary care can provide equivalent care to doctors'. *British Medical Journal*, 324 (2002) 819–824.

10. Department of Health. *Achieving and Sustaining Improved Access to Primary Care.* (2002b). http://www.dh.gov.uk/PolicyAndGuidance/OrganisationPolicy/ PrimaryCare/PrimaryCareTrusts/PrimaryCareTrustsArticle/fs/en?CONTENT_ID =4016138&chk=gvOn07 (accessed 3/4/05).

11. Scottish Executive. *Our National Health: A Short Guide to the Health Plan Working Together for a Healthy, Caring Scotland.* www.scotland.gov.uk/ library3/health/sghp-00.asp (accessed 4/1/06).

12. Kinley J., Hancock, D. and Casterton, J. 'Nurse prescribing in palliative care: Putting training into practice'. *Nurse Prescribing*, 2: 2 (2004) 60–64.

13. Raftery, S. and Elborn, J.S. 'Do nurses do it better?' *Thorax*, 57 (2002) 659–660.

14. Rafferty, J.P., Yao, G.L., Murchie, P., Campbell, N.C. and Ritchie, L.D. 'Cost-effectiveness of nurse-led secondary prevention clinics for coronary

heart disease in primary care: Follow-up of a randomised controlled trial'. *British Medical Journal*, 330 (2005) 707–710.

15. Davis, J. and Hemmingway, S. 'Supplementary prescribing in mental health nursing'. *Nursing Times*, 99: 32 (2003) 28–30.

16. Grant, R. 'Moving forward with supplementary prescribing'. *Prescriber*, 16: 4 (2005). http:www.escriber.com/Prescriber?Features (accessed 30/3/05).

17. Hennell, S.L. 'Competency and the use of clinical management plans in rheumatology in practice'. *Nurse Prescribing*, 2: 1 (2004) 26–30.

18. Bellingham, J. 'How supplementary prescribing is working for pharmacists in practice'. *Prescribing and Medicines Management*, July: (2004) 2–3.

19. Bellingham, J. 'Pharmacists positive about supplementary prescribing'. *Prescribing and Medicines Management*, 6 (2003) 5–6. http://www.pjonline.com/MedicinesManagement (accessed 30/3/05).

20. The National Pharmaceutical Association. 'Chronic disease management'. *Pharmacy Flyer*, Issue 15, Summer (2004). www.npa.co.uk (accessed 30/3/05).

21. Department of Health. *Supplementary Prescribing by Nurses and Pharmacists within the NHS in England: A Guide for Implementation* (London: Crown Copyright, 2003).

22. Department of Health. *Mechanisms for Nurse and Pharmacist Prescribing and Supply of Medicines: Revised* (2004). http://www.dh.gov.uk/assetRoot/04/08/38/92/04083892.pdf (accessed 24/2/05).

23. National prescribing centre. *Supplementary prescribing: A Resource to Help Healthcare Professionals to Understand the Framework and Opportunities* (2003). http://www.npc.co.uk/publications/healthcare_resource.pdf (accessed 24/2/05).

24. Baird, A. 'Supplementary prescribing: One general practice's experience of implementation'. *Nurse Prescribing*, 2: 2 (2004) 72–75.

25. Courtenay, M. 'Supplementary prescribing: What impact will it have?' *Future Prescriber* 5:3 (2004). www.escriber.com/FuturePrescriber/Features (accessed 30/3/05).

26. Hay, A. and Bradley, E. 'Supplementary nurse prescribing'. *Nursing Standard*, 18: 4 (2004) 33–39.

Chapter 4

Government targets: getting the best from non-medical prescribing

Sandy Tinson

Introduction

The introduction of non-medical prescribing into the mainstream of health care provision has been a slow and disappointing milestone for nurses, pharmacists, AHPs and other independent contractors. The NHS has undergone an unprecedented growth in activity and investment since 2000 and it is particularly discouraging to see that the potential of non-medical prescribing is not being harnessed by health care providers. In 2000, the Department of Health set ambitious targets for nurse prescribers and yet the current figure is well short of the predicted 10,000 nurses. In contrast, other targets, for example waiting times and access, have been reached and in some areas surpassed.

This chapter will explore the impact and significance of targets upon the way health care is delivered and how, together with associated initiatives and developments within the NHS, non-medical prescribing can make a substantial contribution to the NHS Plan.[1]

Targets and the NHS Plan

Targets are not a recent phenomenon. There have always been targets and they have provided managers and clinicians alike with clear goals. However, there is certainly more emphasis upon targets in the current political climate. Targets have more usually been regarded as 'carrots', rather than 'sticks', and certainly within the private sector, a target achieved is usually associated with some sort of financial or professional gain. In that respect there are certain similarities between the government targets for health and performance management. The organisations that achieve the targets and thus the required performance measures have the opportunity to apply for Foundation Trust status and in doing so gain a significant increase in autonomy and financial control. Conversely, those organisations that fail to reach targets are penalised and subject to rigorous external review and monitoring processes. At an executive level this can mean that chief executives and board members are dismissed.

Clearly targets are powerful drivers for change and have been responsible for driving forward an ambitious agenda that has resulted in substantial changes in the way health care is delivered. The NHS Plan[1] and more latterly the NHS Improvement Plan[2] have made the greatest impact on the patient experience. Patients no longer wait more than 48 hours for an appointment with their doctor or more than 4 hours in accident and emergency departments. The waiting lists have reduced considerably and patients can soon expect to wait no more than 18 weeks for follow-up appointments in outpatients or for surgery.

There is no doubt that targets promote and support changes to service delivery with a real sense of urgency and in order to achieve these changes, health economies are compelled to work in partnership.

For example, the access and waiting time targets can only realistically be achieved if primary and secondary care services:

- acknowledge the patient pathway
- analyse the interface between organisations/services
- identify how to make best use of the skills of all team members
- identify new and enhanced roles
- improve communication for clinicians and patients.

This basic '5 point plan' can be applied to a wide range of service provision and in providing a clear focus for activity, targets demand that individuals and/or teams work together and thereby gain a clearer understanding of each others' roles and sphere of practice.

Exercise

What specific targets have been set for your specialist area? How do you measure the achievement of targets?

Success and achievement, generally, go hand in hand with target setting and particularly where demonstrable improvements to the delivery and quality of patient care can be quantified. Non-medical prescribing could so easily contribute to the reduction in waiting times, increased access and patient satisfaction and yet currently there is scant evidence to support this premise.[3] It is extremely significant that targets influence commissioning decisions and Primary Care Trusts (PCTs), as commissioners of local health service provision, are therefore both informed and directed by targets and associated performance measures.

Lastly and possibly most significantly, NHS Trust Boards are highly committed to achieving targets, therefore endorsement and support from a trust board cannot be underestimated in terms of influencing the organisation's agenda and future investment plans. Non-medical prescribers can play a key role in meeting some of the more challenging targets. However, their contribution must be clearly articulated and form part of the health economy's strategic direction. Possible barriers and strategies to address them will be considered later within this chapter. Predictably, there is also a downside to the increased emphasis on targets and performance monitoring. It may result in resources and activity being concentrated upon those areas under specific scrutiny or where they will achieve the greatest impact. Organisations may prioritise activity and resources in order to gain the biggest influence upon targets. This may lead to a disjointed and uncoordinated approach to service development. Roles are often developed in isolation, sometimes based on the expertise and interest of individuals already in post. Non-medical prescribing may be considered ideal for one service or specialist area, without consideration of the wider service implications for the future.

Another potential problem arising from quantitative target setting, for example as with the target for 10,000 nurse prescribers,[4] or 3000 community matrons,[5] is that organisations may respond with the required quota of specialists in order to meet the target, without regard for the local health need or specific recruitment issues. There is also a danger that posts will be recruited to without due consideration for future workforce planning needs or succession planning. The pressure within organisations to meet deadlines and targets cannot be overemphasised and there is a real danger that unless there is clear strategic leadership; developments which could enhance both patient care and professional opportunities will fail and lose credibility for the future.

The Challenges of Non-Medical Prescribing

It is clear that the government is committed to the growth of non medical prescribing. It has been high on the national agenda for several years and the important role it can play in achieving improvements in patient care has been highlighted in several key strategic documents[6–10] which support the enhanced role for nurses, allied health professionals and pharmacists.

Exercise

Are you or your colleagues working in enhanced roles? In what way would you or a patient in your care benefit from your being a prescriber?

Although the government appears to be committed to the growth of non-medical prescribing and there are many examples of where it has been well evaluated and has enhanced patient care,[3] it would be fair to say that it has still not been universally embraced by all organisations. There are several reasons for this.

The long and protracted introduction of nurse prescribing over a period of 15 years culminated in the roll-out of a national programme and an extremely limited formulary in 1998. The programme was extremely structured and intended for HVs and DNs only. Practice nurses who were working in general practice at this time were excluded from this programme unless they had previously qualified as a HV or DN. This bureaucratic barrier did little to engage the wider health community to the potential benefits of prescribing.

Disappointingly and perhaps as a consequence of this indiscriminate roll-out, the number of nurses who used their new responsibilities was limited and research has shown that more than 80 per cent were generating three or less prescriptions a week.[11] For detractors, these statistics only reinforce a justification not to commit to non-medical prescribing.

Overall, the process for the introduction of non-medical prescribing has been disjointed, lacking both structure and focus. Underwood[12] believes the piecemeal approach to formulary extension, the initial limitations of the formulary and the disorganised way policy changes are announced have resulted in considerable disappointment and a lack of engagement by both clinicians and managers alike. This somewhat chaotic approach has both frustrated and confused those charged with taking this agenda forward. With each change of policy and direction there is a need to amend current arrangements and provide additional activity and support structures. However, despite each new development there still does not seem to be a clear vision of where or when it will end.

The nature and depth of training has also been identified as a possible reason for a lack of engagement. The training for non-medical prescribing is, by its very nature, intensive and requires adequate mentorship and supervision. Some managers have cited service pressures and the lack of service cover as a deterrent, as they are not able to release staff to attend the training programme. The greatest barrier in some organisations has been the lack of financial support for the medical supervision required.[13] Whilst some GPs and consultants can see the benefits of non-medical prescribing and are willing to support staff, there is a limit to the altruism expected from medical colleagues. This problem has been particularly highlighted in primary care and areas with single-handed GPs, where both resources and time are limited. This may be more of a challenge for the supervision requirements of AHPs and pharmacists, who do not necessarily have the one-to-one relationship with medical colleagues.

The wholesale acceptance of PGDs has also proved to be a disincentive in some areas. The number of PGDs currently in use seems to be increasing rather than decreasing[14] and they are regarded by some clinicians and managers alike as a viable alternative to the introduction of non-medical prescribing. In order to examine the arguments around non-medical prescribing versus PGDs see Chapter 18.

Exercise

Are PGDs used in your area of practice, and if so for what reason? What are the alternatives?

Another fundamental barrier to the introduction of prescribing may be the fears for patient safety raised by some doctors' leaders.[15] The threat to traditional professional boundaries and roles may prove to be a hindrance to those striving to introduce it into their organisation. Devolution and the implementation differences throughout different countries within the United Kingdom also make non-medical prescribing a difficult concept for managers to commit to. See Chapter 1.

Whilst this may offer a possible explanation for the relatively small numbers of non-medical prescribers currently practising in the United Kingdom, there are some practical concerns which have detracted and sometimes overwhelmed the benefits it affords. These included the inability to repeat prescribe, the need to handwrite prescriptions, the problems of prescribing for patients without a GP, lack of clarity around changing doses and a general confusion about what non-medical prescribers can or cannot prescribe and for what conditions. These 'day to day' challenges not only demotivated clinicians and managers but also made it more difficult to take forward the strategic direction. Some of these issues have now been addressed and solutions are either in place or are soon to be so. For instance, computer-generated prescriptions are now available through some of the computerised medical records systems for example EMIS. Nurses and pharmacists are now able to independently prescribe for any condition falling within their competence and supplementary prescribing has become a viable option for those AHPs who are able to access training. The impact is that currently, many of the training programmes for non-medical prescribing are now fully taken up. This may, however, have more to do with the soon-to-be withdrawn government funding that these places afford.

The Integration of Non-Medical Prescribing into Workforce Planning

The NHS Plan[16] set out a national strategy to grow and develop the NHS workforce. Building the necessary workforce capacity requires planning at organisational, local and national levels. Local Delivery Plans (LDP) contribute to this by describing:

- *how* health economies will deliver effective workforce supply, through more staff working differently
- *what* the impact of service developments will be on workforce development and planning.

Workforce planning can be described as the process by which an organisation, under changing conditions, determines its workforce needs and develops plans to address them. Put more simply it means it is the process of getting *the right people, with the right skills, in the right place, in the right jobs at the right time*.

Workforce planning is basically a three-step process which involves:

- identifying the current and future skills and numbers of staff needed to deliver new and improved services
- analysing the current workforce in relation to those needs
- highlighting shortages, surpluses and competency gaps.

This provides the basis for producing a three- to five-year Workforce Development Plan which sets out where staff and skills should be placed to meet the changing needs and priorities of the organisation.

Effective workforce planning should help NHS organisations meet the proposed targets in the NHS Plan, and the ability for the workforce to work in different ways is seen as key to achieving those targets. In fact, 'working differently' is one of two key objectives identified within the NHS Plan.

Whilst many NHS organisations strive to achieve effective and realistic workforce planning, in reality, the outcome is often determined by local recruitment, financial constraints and the need to provide an immediate response to local need.

Non-medical prescribing should be regarded as a key component within current workforce plans. However, this requires a pro-active approach. A strategy for the introduction of non-medical prescribers into the workforce should be developed at least one or two years before they are required. This guarantees they are adequately trained and placed in an area of geographical or clinical practice where there is the greatest need and which will produce the greatest impact.

Exercise

Carry out a SWOT analysis of the implementation of non-medical prescribing in your area of work. What are the implications for the workforce in response to your analysis. Compare this with that in Chapter 16.

Potential independent and supplementary prescribers already exist within the current workforce. They are the nurses, pharmacists, physiotherapists, podiatrists and radiographers who are in service; who can access appropriate training programmes to enable them to prescribe. How they are identified and supported offers yet another challenge.

Workforce planning is not an exact science and within the NHS it has traditionally responded more to a 'quick fix', personal interest and capability rather than the needs of the service. This has the potential to result in clinicians with enhanced skills being situated in those areas of the least need or an overprovision of clinicians with inappropriate skills.

There is a counterbalance to this argument. Jordan and Griffiths[15] believe that as the demand for medical care outweighs supply in many parts of the United Kingdom, there is a danger that non-medical prescribing and other expanded roles will be dispropor-tionately located in areas of economic deprivation.

Both arguments support the view that in order for the full poten-tial to be realised, the workforce plan should clearly reflect the objectives of the organisation and its commitment to the imple-mentation of non-medical prescribing.

There is always the risk that in striving to meet targets in this area, an organisation will choose to go for the short-term response rather than the long-term solution.

In order to successfully integrate non-medical prescribing into workforce planning and development, it calls for clear leadership and an acknowledgement of the resource implications involved in taking forward this change. The investment required cannot be underestimated. However, the long-term benefits will be significant.

Developing the Workforce Now and for the Future

Currently, NHS managers are considering how they can implement new ways of working, with limited resources, in order to achieve maximum gain. It is imperative that the benefits of independent and supplementary prescribing are explicit and seen as central to the provision of new services and the means to achieving targets.

Hopefully, managers and leaders are taking into account the existing workforce, assessing their education and training needs and working with Higher Education Institutions (HEI) and Strategic Health Authorities (SHAs) to see how they can achieve competent and confident practitioners for the future. If they are to learn anything from the past, it would serve them well to re-examine the barriers and benefits already identified during the introduction of non-medical prescribing education and training since around 1995.

Competent prescribing is only one outcome of a much more complex professional development journey. The skills of assessment, diagnosis and treatment, together with knowledge of pharmacology, ethics and legal awareness, should be implicit within pre-registration training. Whilst each professional group may bring another dimension and expertise to the role of prescriber, it is imperative that HEIs support this at the earliest stage possible.

It is fair to say that, at the moment, NHS managers are 'skilling up' individuals within their organisations in areas where it can be demonstrated that prescribing can enhance the patient journey. Whist it is important to do this, it is also necessary to establish how education programmes can enhance the skills of the workforce of the future. This can only be achieved by reviewing current education contracts and adopting a local health economy approach, where prescribing is seen as an integral part of ongoing workforce development.

Currently the education programme for non-medical prescribing is, by its very nature, intensive and expensive and must address the specialist needs of individuals within a multi-disciplinary programme; therefore the need for an established foundation programme for all professional groups is vital.

Established programmes of CPD are also essential, to ensure that ongoing quality and standards are maintained. NHS organisations must consider how this is to be provided and by whom. Each organisation should have a prescribing lead in place but the scope and responsibility of this role is variable and may result in inequitable support programmes across organisations, sometimes within the same health economy. PCTs, until 2006 were much smaller organisations than their acute and mental health counterparts and it is possible that the capacity and capability of individual PCTs impacted on their ability to provide the necessary level of support to non-medical prescribers. Likewise, the introduction of non-medical prescribing was slower in some larger acute and mental health hospitals and there may not have been the viability or volume of staff to warrant a specific CPD programme. This too is changing now that the restrictions on prescribing have largely been lifted from nurses and pharmacists and now that AHPs are availing themselves of supplementary prescribing skills.

A whole system approach, which gains maximum benefit from education contracts, would be the ideal answer. The benefits are twofold: not only does this provide a viable and economic solution but it also fosters interprofessional and cross-boundary working. See Chapter 19 for more on CPD in relation to prescribing.

Grasping the Opportunity

Never has there been a time when non-medical prescribing has such an important role to play in future health care planning. The extensive modernisation agenda, together with reforms in the way primary care is delivered,[17-19] has provided managers with an ideal opportunity to embed non-medical prescribing within service and role redesign.

The Changing Face of Primary Care

The delivery of primary care has been influenced in several ways. These include:

▷ **The nGMS Contract**

The most significant developments within primary care have been the introduction of Personal Medical Services (PMS) and the new General Medical Services contract (nGMS).[17,18] Medical practitioners are no longer paid for items of service but for a package of services which they provide to their practice population. Practices can also provide Local Enhanced Services (LES) which makes it possible to offer a service above and beyond the requirement of the nGMS contract. In many instances it is other professionals who are better placed, rather than doctors, to provide that service. The ability to prescribe can only enhance the development of such innovations.

▷ **Out of Hours Service**

Another significant development arising from the nGMS contract is the arrangements for out of hours. Formerly the responsibility of GPs alone, this transferred to the PCTs since January 2005. In some areas, nurses, pharmacists and some AHPs have been integrated into this service and this extended role can realistically enhance and benefit urgent care to patients.

▷ **The Pharmacy Contract**

The Pharmacy Contract, introduced in April 2005, sets out clear requirements for community pharmacists which could clearly embrace and benefit from pharmacists being able to prescribe.

New Roles

▷ **The Community Matron**

The community matron is both a target in itself and having targets set as part of the role. The target is for 3000 community matrons to be employed by 2007 who will reduce bed occupancy of those with chronic conditions by 20 per cent in the first year.[5] See Chapter 11.

New Services

▷ **Management of Long-term Conditions**

There are real benefits to the patient with a long-term condition whose medicines can be managed and monitored by a nurse or pharmacist and should form part of an organisation's strategic development and support the organisation's target to reduce in patient 'bed days' for these patients.

▶ **Minor Ailments, Minor Injury Clinics and NHS Walk-in Centres**
These are integral to improving access for patients and are invariably run without a doctor on the premises. Their contribution to the reduction in waiting times and increased access cannot be underestimated. See Chapter 5.

▶ **Family Planning**
Both nurses and pharmacists have a part to play in meeting the government targets for reducing teenage pregnancy and non-medical prescribing can augment that service.

Case study

One PCT with a diverse population and disparate health needs implemented a service for those 'hard to reach' clients who may not register with a GP or do not readily access traditional health services, such as asylum seekers, drug users, street workers or the homeless. A nurse-led PMS project was established in 2004.

Two nurses, who were already prescribers, provide a range of services to these clients including:

▶ a sexual health clinic
▶ a minor ailments/injuries unit
▶ a child health clinic
▶ long-term conditions management.

It provides a viable and sometimes preferable alternative to GP services where patients can be assessed, diagnosed and treated (or referred as appropriate) on site. The benefits are that patients are satisfied and emergency admissions are averted. National and local targets for teenage pregnancy, sexual health and drug management are met and it provides a tangible and effective example of how inequalities are being addressed within the town. Most significantly it has shown how the enhanced role can afford real benefits for patients.

Taking the Agenda Forward

There would never seem to be a better time to grasp the opportunities which will ensure non-medical prescribing is seen as integral to future workforce planning and service redesign. However, in order for it to make a difference and have a significant impact on targets, it requires a high level of commitment from trust boards and executive teams and a reassurance of an integrated approach to the implementation across the organisation and patient pathways.

It would be fair to say that, for many NHS managers, the implementation has, up until recently, been localised and small scale. Its potential has not been fully realised and has not yet reached the consciousness of many decision-makers. The latest legislative changes are wide-ranging and so this situation is changing as organisations see the benefits, not only for patients but for themselves and their ability to meet challenging government targets. However, it is the responsibility of individuals, teams and clinical leaders to ensure barriers are removed and a proactive approach to non-medical prescribing is adopted across the whole health care economy.

References

1. DH. *The NHS Plan: A Plan for Investment, A Plan for Reform.* Gateway reference (London: Crown Copyright, July 2000).

2. DH. *The NHS Improvement Plan: Putting People at the Heart of Public Services.* Gateway reference 3398 (London: Crown Copyright, 2004).

3. Latter, S. and Courtenay, M. 'Effectiveness of nurse prescribing'. *Journal of Clinical Nursing,* 13 (2003) 26–32.

4. DH. *Consultation on Proposals to Extend Nurse Prescribing.* Gateway reference (London: Crown Copyright, October 2000).

5. John Reid, Health Secretary; House of Commons statement, 24 June 2004.

6. DH. *Making a Difference: Strengthening the Nursing, Midwifery and Health Visiting Contribution to Health and Health care* (London: Crown Copyright, 1999).

7. DH. Chief Nursing Officer. *Implementing the NHS Plan: Ten Key Roles for Nurses. Professional Letter.* Gateway reference (London: Crown Copyright, November 2002).

8. DH. *Liberating the Talents: Helping Primary Care Trusts and Nurses to Deliver the NHS Plan*. Gateway reference (London: Crown Copyright, November 2002).

9. DH. *Launch of the Ten High Impact Changes for Service Improvement and Delivery*. Gateway reference 3483 (London: Crown Copyright, September 2004).

10. DH. *Extending Independent Nurse Prescribing within the NHS in England: A Guide for Implementation*. Gateway reference 2783 (London: Crown Copyright, February 2004).

11. While, A. and Biggs, K. 'Benefits and challenges of nurse prescribing'. *Journal of Advanced Nursing*, 6 (2004) 559–567.

12. Underwood, F. 'Supporting and developing new nurse prescribers in secondary care'. *Nurse Prescribing*, 2: 6 (2004) 256–260.

13. Lewis, C. 'The late show'. *Health Service Journal*, 8 April (2004) 28–29.

14. Green, H. 'Nurse prescribing in the acute sector: One trust's perspective'. *Nurse Prescribing*, 2: 1 (2004) 9–14.

15. Jordan, S. and Griffiths, H. 'Nurse Prescribing: Developing the evaluation agenda'. *Nursing Standard*, 18: 29 (2004) 40–44.

16. DH. *HR in the NHS Plan: More Staff Working Differently*. Gateway reference (London: Crown Copyright, July 2002).

17. DH. *The NHS (GMS Contract) Regulation 2004*. Statutory instrument (2004) No. 291.

18. DH. *The NHS (PMS) (miscellaneous amendments) Regulation 2004*. Statutory instrument (2004) No. 2694.

19. DH. *Practice Based Commissioning: Promoting clinical engagement*. Gateway reference 4301 (London: Crown Copyright, December 2004).

Part II

Nursing and midwifery perspectives on independent and supplementary prescribing

Chapter 5

Walk-in centre perspectives

Ruth Lonsdale

Introduction

Walk-in centres (WICs) were set up in England as a response to changing demands within the health service. It was envisaged that patients should be able to see a primary health care professional within one day and a GP within two days of request. Everyone attending Accident and Emergency Departments should be seen within 4 hours.[1] Patients also needed to be given a choice of when to be seen and the extended opening hours of WICs addressed this need. The NHS plan[1] had five aims that WICs would contribute towards meeting in relation to the overall strategy. See Table 5.1.

Table 5.1 Main aims of NHS Plan[1]

Aims	Outcomes
Partnership	Making all parts of the health and social care system work better together with the right emphasis at each care level
Performance	Improve both clinical performance and health service productivity
Professionals	Increased flexibility in training and working practice; remove demarcation in terms of roles
Patient care	Fast and convenient access to services Patients to be involved in their own care
Prevention	Tackling inequalities and focussing on addressing the causes of avoidable ill health

According to Salisbury et al.[2] WICs were developed in order to achieve the following:

- improved access for care – achieved by providing care at a more convenient time, in a more convenient location, with minimal waiting;
- reducing demand on other NHS services, thus maximising efficiency;
- providing safe, high quality care by nurses with decision-support software;
- increased appropriateness of patients seen by other NHS providers – achieved by nurses encouraging self-care and helping patients identify when they need to consult a doctor.

Walk-in centres are ideally placed to treat patients who are not registered with GPs such as the homeless, tourists and asylum seekers who otherwise would end up attending Accident and Emergency Departments. They have contributed to the overall success of the health service as these aims have been met. On average 84 per cent of patients see a GP within 2 days and 77 per cent of patients attending Accident and Emergency Departments are seen within 4 hours.[3]

By May 2005, a total of 66 WICs had opened, with many more planned. Including Accident and Emergency Departments, these WICs have been situated in convenient locations and in town centres. In order to make services more convenient and easily accessible for patients, no appointments are necessary and the opening hours of the centres are early morning to late evening (usually 7 a.m. to 10 p.m.), 365 days a year, as determined by the Department of Health.[4]

Experienced nurses from a wide range of backgrounds including paediatrics, accident and emergency and community nursing initially staffed the centres. Computer assisted software (CAS) was installed nationally in all WICs, to aid diagnosis and give confidence to both staff and patients. New WICs no longer have to have CAS systems. This reflects the expertise of nurses working in WICs. To fulfil the role of a WIC nurse, one needs to be able to practise autonomously and take responsibility for the diagnosis, management and discharge of patients.[5]

Exercise

Consider the location of your nearest WIC or similar service. What population does it serve? What services does it provide? If the service was unavailable what would the alternatives be?

By August 2001, an average of 2556 patients attended a WIC per month with the number of visits rising.[2,6] Among the commonest reasons for consultation were blood pressure checks, viral illnesses, patients requesting emergency contraception, minor illnesses and dressings. Table 5.2 shows the top 20 reasons for attendance.[6]

Table 5.2 gives a snapshot of the types of conditions patients present with in WICs nationally, for advice and treatment.[6]

Table 5.2 Top 20 reasons for Walk-in Centre attendance[6]

Condition	Number attending
Blood pressure check	744
Blocked ears	681
Skin conditions	667
Ear, nose and throat ailments	636
Return dressing	634
Flu or systemic viral infection	578
Other musculoskeletal conditions	577
Unprotected sexual intercourse	513
Other eye conditions	441
Common cold	391
Urinary tract infection	372
Stye, conjunctivitis, blepharitis	372
Tonsillitis or pharyngitis	336
Non-acute wound care	326
Soft tissue injury of ankle, foot or toe	289
Back pain	282
Muscle pain	263
Otitis media	262
Other wounds, soft tissue infection, burns	249
Minor head injury	240

Source: British Medical Journal, 324 (2002) 399–402. Reproduced with permission from the BMJ Publishing Group.

Importantly it was found that 78 per cent of consultations were managed by WIC staff without referral elsewhere. The national findings are not necessarily applicable to all WICs. Different centres will have different patient populations attending and in the author's experience, not many patients attend for blood pressure monitoring but with more general conditions such as viral infections, accidents and for emergency contraception.

Exercise

Consider the range of conditions listed in Table 5.2. Select one or two conditions from the list that you would be likely to come across in practice. Write up a simulated consultation using history taking skills and consider the differential diagnoses and potential treatments. Take account of both prescribing and non-prescribing decisions. If you would prescribe, make a brief note of the evidence you used to formulate your decision.

Ear Wax

The second highest reason for attendance according to Table 5.2 is 'blocked ears'; however, Salisbury et al.[6] have not discussed what this actually means. Usually it implies that the patient has hardened wax and has presented with difficulty in hearing. This condition is more common in the elderly and in those who wear hearing aids or use cotton buds.[7] Where ear wax is causing problems such as deafness the prescriber will usually give a prescription for olive oil ear drops, sodium bicarbonate drops or advise the patient to buy them, with advice on administration. Differential diagnoses include otitis externa, which may be treated with antibiotics by the nurse prescriber, and foreign bodies, which the nurse might suspect in children. Diagnosis is made from clinical history and by examination of the ear canal with an auroscope. Ear irrigation is much less common than it used to be due to the dangers of perforation. Electronic irrigators are much safer than syringes as they control the water pressure and direction of flow.[8] Nurses should be trained in ear irrigation and be able to identify contraindications and cautions.

Case study 1

A 25 year old woman presented to a WIC with a history of earache with itching for 2 days. During discussion it became apparent that the patient had no signs and symptoms other than ear pain. A differential diagnosis was made, which on examination would be confirmed or refuted. Consent was obtained for examination of both ears. The left ear had no sign of infection but the right tragus was painful to touch and on moving the pinna the patient experienced pain. The external auditory canal was dry, flaky and red. The tympanic membrane was clearly visible as was the handle of the malleus. A diagnosis of acute otitis externa was made with a diagnosis of chronic otitis externa being refuted on the basis of clinical history. Due to the presence of eczematous inflammation a prescription was given for Otomize ear spray 1 original pack (generic prescribing is usually undertaken but where there are combined ingredients, it is sometimes clearer for the pharmacist if a brand name is used). The dose was to apply 1 metered spray into the ear 3 times daily for 7 days. Should symptoms get worse or show no improvement the patient was advised to return for review.

Otomize ear spray contains:

- ▶ dexamethasone 0.1 per cent – topical corticosteroid to treat eczema
- ▶ neomycin sulphate 3250 units/ml – topical anti infective
- ▶ glacial acetic acid 2 per cent – antifungal and antibacterial[9]

At the time of writing, suitably qualified nurses are able to prescribe from the BNF for any condition falling within the nurses' competence. Nurses working as independent prescribers in WICs can reduce waiting times for patients. The literature states that nurse prescribers ensure treatments are initiated speedily as a result of prescribing and patients will take advantage of the easy access provided.[10]

Patient Group Directions (PGDs) in Walk-in Centres

First level nurses working in WICs can operate under PGDs. For a definition of PGD, see Chapter 18. Normally training and assessment is provided for all WIC nurses prior to them issuing medication. There is no common training available and the standard differs in various WICs. Some WICs will have pharmacist input into the training, others will use nurse clinicians and some will use senior nurses. However, all receive training and assessment of competence according to local policies. The senior nurse will maintain a register of staff who have trained and the medicines they can issue. Nurses sign to say that they understand and agree to work within a specific PGD. Salisbury et al.[2] found that the standard of PGDs for issuing antibiotics in WICs was variable, with some not meeting the legal requirements. This raises some concerns about the use of PGDs in practice. In addition, record keeping in relation to PGDs was found to be inadequate. It may be that the training in the use of PGDs needs to be more rigorous as it is for independent and supplementary prescribing.

Local policies can differ, but first level nurses demonstrating the necessary knowledge and competence to administer medicines are professionally accountable for their actions.[11] In some areas specialist training is updated annually. Other areas will manage standards locally, by auditing patient records on a regular basis. Outside agencies such as the Department of Health can ask for monitoring of records in relation to medicines issued under PGDs. This helps them to understand the changing workload of WICs.

Exercise

Audit is used extensively throughout the Health Service. Have you been involved in an audit and, if yes, for what purpose? How were the results disseminated? Carry out a short audit of your prescribing habits (or those where you work), highlighting frequently prescribed medicines/products and rationalise why this is so. Is this best practice?

In a WIC, one can see the benefit of nurses being able to use both PGDs and independent prescribing because of the way in which these systems complement each other for the benefit of patients. It may not be appropriate to train all nurses working in WICs to become independent prescribers.

Whether the nurse supplies, administers or prescribes medication, records must be adequately maintained.[11] For nurses who supply and/or administer, the details should be recorded in the patient records as follows:

▶ date of supply and/or administration
▶ name of the medicine

- batch number
- expiry date
- any adverse reaction.

The GP practice is informed of any medicines prescribed. The initial computer system in WICs did not provide the detailed records that would be available in general practice and therefore nurses who prescribed needed to find out what other medicines patients were taking and set up audit systems to track prescriptions given. Carbon copied notepads could be used. As a result of gathering this information the nurse prescribers could see what medicines needed to be prescribed regularly and those of limited use. Their non-prescribing colleagues who needed to issue under PGD could benefit from this system because the frequently used prescribed medicines could be 'converted' into a PGD where appropriate.

Table 5.3 shows the information that is required on the label of medicines issued under a PGD. This information must be included in all cases.

For independent prescribing a prescription is completed for each patient following the 12 principles of writing a prescription (see Appendix 3).

Patients who attend WICs should be seen by one member of staff who will, in most cases, be able to complete the whole episode of care including supply or prescription of medicines. Not all episodes of care in WICs can be completed because the patient may attend with problems that necessitate hospital admission, accident and emergency referral or referral to a GP for further assessment. When the WICs first opened, responsibility lay with the Department

Table 5.3 Information required on pharmaceutical label when issuing medicines under a PGD[12]

Patient information	Medicine information	Centre information
Name	Name	Name of issuing centre
Date of Birth	Dose	Date of Issue
	Route of administration	
	Frequency	

Source: Health Service Circular 2000/026, © Crown Copyright, 2006.

of Health for the standard of care provided and the budgeting processes. Now that WICs are established, this responsibility has been passed to the individual employing organisations to ensure the budget is adequate for service provision.[13]

Quality Control Issues

Each Trust has a duty of care regarding quality in respect of The Health Act.[14] It states that it is the duty of each Health Authority, PCT and Acute NHS Trust to put and keep in place arrangements for monitoring and improving the quality of health care provided to individuals. This ensures that patients do receive a high level of care but also that systems are in place to support staff especially when advanced roles such as independent prescribing are undertaken. Structured formal clinical supervision is a way of ensuring that this happens. *Clinical supervision* has been described as:

> a formal process of professional support and learning which enables individual practitioners to develop knowledge and competence, assume responsibility for their own practice and enhance consumer protection and safety of care in complex clinical situations.[15]

Clinical supervision in this setting means sitting with peers in a formal and confidential setting, presenting case reviews. Support, challenge and discussion take place. Learning outcomes will be given at the end so that learning is enhanced and the scope of practice can be widened. Reflection occurs on care delivery, and the detailed consultation is analysed. Some WICs encourage teams to have the occasional day away for team building. In order for this type of supervision to work well, it needs to be undertaken within a team where members feel safe and where there is an atmosphere of trust. For nurses who prescribe, this gives an excellent opportunity to discuss the impact of prescribing on their roles as well as gaining knowledge from others and for updating. See Chapter 19 for information on continuing professional development.

For the new nurse prescriber, support will be needed from colleagues. Writing a prescription gives more autonomy but with that comes more responsibility. Support may be needed as it is a new role, and there are often time delays in registration with the NMC and for the prescription pads to arrive.

Exercise

Think about the statements made in relation to clinical supervision. How will/do you keep up to date with prescribing issues and ensure that you maintain a responsible approach to this area of practice?

Clinical Issues

There are many opportunities within WICs to undertake episodes of care, which mean that the practitioner will need to make a holistic assessment, diagnose, treat and provide 'safety netting' for each patient. 'Safety netting' is described as catering for the 'worst case scenario'.[16] In relation to prescribing, a diagnosis and management plan will be implemented but should unforeseen problems occur, the patient is informed of when and how to seek further help. There are many opportunities to practise as an independent prescriber in WICs.

Practitioners work autonomously and independently but they are also part of a team. Team members value one another's expertise and are willing to learn from each other in order to provide best practice to patients. The team concept is enabling and empowering, allowing the practitioner to learn new knowledge and skills. Working with uncertainty is a challenge.

Medication can be prescribed for certain illnesses only by qualified nurse prescribers. Not all nurses in WICs are prescribers and the range of PGDs is limited. The public do not necessarily understand why one nurse can write a prescription and another cannot. The recent expansion of independent nurse prescribing has been welcome.

Other Presentations in WICs

Patients with skin conditions attend WICs. Prescribing for eczema can be carried out but care should be taken as nurses are not there to take on a caseload role. Those attending the centres will be treated until the next prescription only as they remain under the care of a GP. Prescribing will include emollients and topical corticosteroids if needed.

Parents may present with children who have viral illnesses such as chickenpox. Health advice is given in relation to how to treat the child and the need for avoiding pregnant women especially in the first and last trimesters as the virus can be harmful to the unborn fetus. Children are normally well in these instances but advice is given in relation to the child worsening. Advice can be given regarding the use of treatments such as calamine lotion to relieve itching.

Patients attend with other viral illnesses, commonly sore throats and influenza. The challenge to the nurse prescriber is in the educational role and discussing with patients that antibiotics are not necessary.[17,18] This can only be achieved once a thorough examination has been conducted. Prescriptions for items such as paracetamol and ibuprofen can be more costly to patients who pay for prescriptions as they are generally cheaper to buy over the counter and most patients would be advised to do so. Patients with tonsillitis can be treated with antibiotics, however, the nurse independent prescriber may prefer to diagnose tonsillitis, exclude quinzy and glandular fever and prescribe or advise on use of analgesia, along with patient advice about the self-limiting nature of tonsillitis.[19]

Due to the long opening times and accessibility of WICs, many patients use them for emergency contraception. Within society there is a need to prevent unwanted pregnancies and therefore Levonelle-2 can be issued under PGD or prescribed. Some nurses are trained in family planning and would like to prescribe contraception in the normal context rather than for emergency purposes. This is within their scope of practice; however, it is wise to consider the wider implications for offering such a service. Those patients who attend general practice or family planning clinics will be offered the full range of women's health services such as cervical cytology screening whereas in WICs these services are not provided. Patients do not always return, therefore the opportunity of follow-up, which is a necessary provision, may be lost. Ethically, if a patient has not managed to get to the practice or clinic to renew the contraceptive pill the nurse prescriber should suggest they go to their local pharmacist or write out a prescription as it is in the patients' best interest to have the medicine. The prescriber can only do this if it is within his or her competence.

Urinary tract infections, too, are common. When a person presents with a urinary tract infection an appropriate antibiotic can be prescribed.

Conjunctivitis (Acute Infective)

An acute infection of the conjunctiva of one or both the eyes accounts for about 35 per cent of eye problems seen in general practice.[20]

Presentation consists of:

- burning or gritty eyes, with minimal pain
- mild photophobia (not always present)
- eyes sticking together on waking
- blurred vision from discharge.

Differential Diagnoses[21]

- Viral conjunctivitis – eyes do not usually stick together, itchy, previous history of conjunctivitis.
- Allergic conjunctivitis – tends to present with itchy eyes, oedema of upper eyelids, in person who suffers from other allergic conditions for example eczema, asthma, allergic rhinitis.
- Irritant conjunctivitis – usually secondary to foreign body for example eyelash, dust other irritants include shampoos or chlorine.
- Acute glaucoma – characterised by severe pain, headache, blurred vision. Examination would reveal diminished vision, hazy cornea, fixed dilated pupil, eye is hard and tender, injection of the sclera.
- Keratitis – unilateral, painful photophobic, injected eye with ciliary injection, corneal ulceration, vision may be affected.
- Iritis – pain and watery eye with ciliary injection; may have fixed, dilated or distorted pupil, headache (not always present).

History and Examination

History is important to exclude other causes of conjunctivitis and other eye problems. Examination reveals a red eye and discharge (purulent or watery). Examination will exclude other conditions whilst confirming diagnosis of infective conjunctivitis. If a more serious diagnosis is suspected the patient would be referred to an eye casualty.

Treatment

Antibiotic use is controversial as 64 per cent of people show clinical remission by 5 days following placebo.[22] However, antibiotic use does improve remission rates by 30 per cent at days 2–5.[23] If present for more than a few days it is often treated with antibiotic eye drops or ointment, along with advice regarding hygiene and not to wear contact lenses until condition is resolved.[21] Eye swab is taken if infection fails to respond to treatment.

Case study 2

A 10-year-old girl attended a WIC accompanied by her mother. She had been rubbing her eyes for three days stating that there was a green discharge and she felt like there was grit in her eyes. She was otherwise well and her mother stated that she had no other problems with her health. Visual acuity testing was carried out to ensure normality of vision. An ophthalmoscope was used to inspect the eyelids, lashes, sclera and pupils. No problems were noted on the eyelids or lashes. Both pupils were equal and reacting to light to which the girl was not sensitive. Both sclera were red with vein injection and there was evidence of green discharge. A diagnosis of bilateral infective conjunctivitis was made. A prescription was given for chloramphenicol ointment 4 g, two tubes to be applied 3–4 times daily and continued for 48 hours after healing. Other advices given when prescribing eye ointment can be seen in Table 5.4.

Table 5.4 General advice given when prescribing eye ointment

	Advice
Hygiene measures	Wash hands before and after touching eyes, use own towel and flannel as the condition is very contagious. Wash each eye separately from the corner outwards
Administration of the dose	Ensure one tube is used for each eye. The pharmacy will label the tubes left and right eyes respectively. Do not exceed stated dose
Storage	Follow the manufacturer's instructions
Pain/discomfort	Do not rub the eyes
Adverse reaction	Stop taking the ointment, follow manufacturer's instructions

Conclusion

Statistics related to WIC attendance demonstrate that patients are very satisfied with the level of care[24] and appreciate that medicines are now available via the nurse prescriber. This service complements the care given in other areas such as general practice or Accident and Emergency Departments. Prescribing is, and will continue to be, an inherent part of the toolkit nurses working within WICs need in order to provide a fast and efficient quality service to the patients attending.

References

1. DH. *The NHS Plan: A Plan for Investment, a Plan for Reform* (London: HMSO, 2000).

2. Salisbury, C., Chalder, M., Scott, T.M., Pope, C. and Moore, L. *National Evaluation of NHS Walk in Centres.* Division of Primary Health Care, University of Bristol, 2000.

3. DH. *The NHS Plan: A Progress Report* (London: HMSO, 2003).

4. DH. *Pioneering NHS Walk in Centres Open.* A Health Service Circular. Reference (1999/116).

5. Rosen, R. and Mountford, L. Developing and supporting extended nursing roles: The challenges of NHS Walk in Centres. *Journal of Advanced Nursing,* 39: 3 (2002) 241–248.

6. Salisbury, C., Chalder, M., Scott, T.M., Pope, C. and Moore, L. What is the role of Walk in Centres in the NHS? *British Medical Journal,* 324 (2002) 399–402.

7. Aung, T. and Mulley, G. Removal of ear wax: 10 minute consultation. *British Medical Journal,* 325 (2002) 27–28.

8. Prodigy. *Prodigy Guidance: Ear wax.* 2nd edition (London: The Stationary Office, 2005).

9. British Medical Association/Royal Pharmaceutical Society of Great Britain. *British National Formulary* (London: BMA/RPSGB, September 2005).

10. Venning, P., Durie, A., Roland, M., Roberts, C. and Leese, B. Randomised controlled trial comparing cost effectiveness of general practitioners and nurse practitioners in primary care. *British Medical Journal,* 320 (2000) 1048–1053.

11. NMC. *Guidelines for Administration of Medicines* (London: NMC, 2004).

12. DH. *Patient Group Directions* (England only) HSC 2000/026 (London: DH, 2000).

13. DH. *Primary Care Prescribing and Budget Setting* (2005) http://www.dh.gov.uk accessed 7/6/05.

14. DH. *The Health Act* (London: The Stationary Office, 1999).

15. DH. *A Vision for the Future: Report of the Chief Nursing Officer* (London: The Stationary Office, 1993).

16. Neighbour, R. *The Inner Consultation: How to Develop an Effective and Intuitive Consulting Style.* 2nd edition (Oxford: Radcliffe Publishing, 1987).

17. Zwart, S., Rovers, Maroeska M., de Melker, Ruut A., emeritus H. and Arno W. Penicillin for acute sore throat in children: Randomised, double blind trial. *British Medical Journal,* 327 (2003) 1324.

18. Little, P., Williamson, I., Warner, G., Gould, C., Gantley, M. and Kinnmonth, A. Open randomised trial of prescribing strategies in managing sore throat. *British Medical Journal,* 314 (1997) 722–727.

19. Thomas, M., Del Mar, C. and Glasziou, P. How effective are treatments other than antibiotics for acute sore throat? *British Journal of General Practice,* 50: 459 (2000) 817–820.

20. Royal College of General Practitioners/Royal College of Ophthalmologists. *Ophthalmology for General Practitioner Trainees* (London: Medical Protection Society, 2001).

21. Prodigy. *Prodigy guidance: Infective conjunctivitis.* 2nd edition (London: The Stationary Office, 2005).

22. Sheikh, A. and Hurwitz, B. Topical antibiotics for acute bacterial conjunctivitis: A systematic review. *British Journal of General Practice,* 51: 467 (2001) 473–477.

23. Everett, H. and Little, P. How do GP's diagnose and manage acute infective conjunctivitis? *Family Practice,* 19: 6 (2002) 658–660.

24. Salisbury C., Manku-Cott, T., Moore, L., Chalder, M. and Sharp, M. Questionnaire survey of users of NHS WIC: observational study. *British Journal of General Practice,* 52: 480 (July 2002) 534–560.

Chapter 6

District nursing perspectives

Sue Dundon and Dawn Brookes

Introduction

This chapter will discuss the role of the district nurse (DN) in relation to prescribing. It will describe the value of non-medical prescribing with particular reference to wound care, dermatology, hypertension and palliative care. The chapter will demonstrate the limitations of the Nurse Prescribing Formulary for Community Practitioners (NPF). Additionally the development of Clinical Management Plans (CMP) through partnerships with general practitioners (GPs) will be addressed. The authors have chosen to use the title 'independent prescriber' (V300) in order to differentiate from that of 'Community Nurse Prescriber' (V100).*

District Nursing

Patients seen by district nursing teams are usually housebound and therefore in need of nursing care in their own home. This may be in residential or sheltered housing as well as privately owned and tenancy housing. Historically, some district nurses have not seen patients in nursing homes but their specialist skills are often required by patients living in these settings. District nurses are beginning to bring their expertise into such environments, including teaching and training of nursing home staff. For the majority of district nurses the patient group seen is elderly. They

---

* See Chapter 2.

may also see patients who have a disability or who require palliative care as well as supporting some patients' early discharge from hospital, for example post-operatively. The types of conditions patients most commonly present with are listed below but the list is by no means exhaustive:

- wounds (trauma, post-operative, decubitis (pressure) ulcers, burns)
- Leg ulcers
- Illnesses requiring palliative care (frequently cancer)
- general debility from ageing (frail, unstable medical conditions, cognitive impairment)
- genito-urinary problems, for example incontinence, retention of urine
- disability, for example motor neurone disease (MND) or multiple sclerosis (MS)
- Long-term conditions, for example Type-2 diabetes mellitus, chronic obstructive pulmonary disease (COPD)
- intravenous therapy including maintenance of special intravenous lines, for example Hickmann lines, peripherally inserted central catheter (PICC) lines
- cytotoxic chemotherapy for cancer
- radiotherapy
- continuous ambulatory peritoneal dialysis (CAPD) for renal failure
- bowel problems, for example constipation
- falls and loss of mobility
- dermatological conditions, for example contact dermatitis, atopic dermatitis.

Exercise

The role of the DN team is changing and there is a necessity for skills to be updated in order to be competent to adopt new roles. In what way will independent prescribing enable the team to provide greater satisfaction for patients? Looking at the list above, make a note of the medicines or other products that a district nurse might need to prescribe which are not listed in the NPF.

Wound Care

Good wound care requires a thorough assessment[1] and a holistic approach. The size, position and state of the wound, for example sloughy or granulating should be described and documented. Photographs taken following informed consent provide a useful baseline. The exudate, pain and any infection are taken into account prior to prescribing a wound dressing. The patient must also be asked if they have any allergies or previous sensitivities to any products or medicines. A full medical and social history including prescribed and over-the-counter medications should be included as part of the assessment. The wound dressing prescribed must be appropriate to facilitate wound healing. The prescription is documented in the patient's notes at home immediately and in those in the GP surgery as soon as possible following the visit and within 24 hours except for bank holidays or weekends when the period may be extended.[2]

Table 6.1 shows the limitations of the NPF compared to independent nurse prescribing.

Table 6.1 Products and indications for wound care products from different formularies

District nurse and health visiting formulary (NPF)	Indications	Nurse independent prescribers
Alginates Film dressings Foam dressings Hydrocolloids Hydrogels	Moderate/heavy exuding wounds Minor abrasions or protection of 'at risk' skin Absorbing exudates and maintaining moisture Lightly to moderately exuding wounds (not usually diabetic wounds)[3] Necrotic or dry sloughy wound (used with caution in diabetic wounds),[3] anaerobic infection, malodorous fungating wounds, wounds requiring anti-microbials and burns	Full range of items listed in the British National Formulary (BNF). For example Metronidazole gel, Silver sulfadiazine 1%

The differences between the NPF and the BNF are enormous and many wounds, particularly leg ulcers have microbes present and the use of topical silver containing dressings is becoming common practice and these have been shown to prevent and even treat wound infections.[4]

Case study

A 75-year-old man who developed a leg ulcer wound infection had been treated with numerous courses of antibiotics over a 2-year period and a wound swab demonstrated that the multiple bacteria present were antibiotic resistant. The options for treatment were limited but included intravenous (IV) antibiotics. The patient was reluctant to be admitted to hospital for treatment and following discussions with him silver sulfadiazine 1 per cent was prescribed by the independent-prescribing district nurse (see Figure 6.1a,b,c). This treatment was commenced on a Friday afternoon when a GP was not available. Treatment would have been delayed by 3 days had the district nurse not been an independent prescriber or the patient may have been admitted to hospital for IV therapy as the wound was rapidly deteriorating and the patient was demonstrating systemic signs of infection.

The wound improved and a later wound swab revealed normal skin flora present and no further infection.

(a)　　　　　　　　　　(b)　　　　　　　　　　(c)

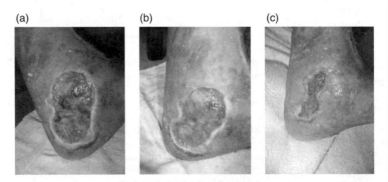

Figure 6.1 (a) Wound infection day 1, (b) and (c) Following topical treatment silver sulfadiazine 1 per cent (© Photos Dawn Brookes)

Exercise

Reflect on this scenario in relation to your own practice. On what evidence would you initiate treatment? If this patient had required IV antibiotics would the nursing team have been able to provide care for the patient at home?

Fears over whether nurses are more likely to prescribe antibiotics resulting in even more antibiotic resistance are largely unfounded. Current practice demonstrates that when an antibiotic is requested for a wound infection or cellulitis, the GP will issue a prescription, more often than not without seeing the patient. Many district nurses discourage patients from the overuse of antibiotics and only request them for use when clinically indicated. The authors have often been in situations where they would not have prescribed antibiotics but a visiting GP will succumb to patient pressure, especially where the patient is not known to them. The district nurse is in an ideal position to determine whether a wound is deteriorating and can usually assess and diagnose the cause. Nevertheless it is important that nurses prescribe within and maintain their professional competence (see Chapter 19).[5] In order to prescribe effectively and safely, the nurse must use evidence-based knowledge.[6,7]

Eczema/Dermatitis

The nurse independent prescriber can prescribe for a range of skin conditions depending on their competence and experience. Eczema (also known as 'dermatitis') is an inflammatory disorder of the skin. The condition can be classified as exogenous (from without), endogenous (from within)[8] or unclassified[9] and, whilst common in children, can be present in adults.[8]

Treatment for dermatitis includes avoiding irritants and triggers such as the house dust mite or pets (Box 6.1). The house dust mite is a common irritant in allergies such as contact dermatitis and often patients require advice regarding avoidance and the use of high washing temperatures of bedding and pillows (over 60 degrees) where this is a factor.

Box 6.1   Common trigger factors for eczema

▶ Family history
▶ Diet/milk
▶ Central heating
▶ House dust mite
▶ Soap
▶ Detergents/perfume
▶ Pets
▶ Clothes for example wool.

Dermatitis can be treated with emollients and/or topical corticosteroids.[10] Wet wrapping is a technique consisting of the use of a warm wet tubular bandage or garment covered by a dry layer of the same. Emollients and topical corticosteroids (where indicated) are applied to the skin prior to the bandage or garment being put in place. Many patients find the treatment beneficial, and advice and prescriptions can be given to people who may gain relief from this treatment as shown in Box 6.2. Wet wrapping[9,11] is commonly used to treat babies and young children but it can be equally effective in soothing symptoms and preventing itching in the elderly patient. Topical corticosteroids can be used under wet wrapping but their absorption is hastened and potent corticosteroids are not recommended when the technique is used.[12] District

---

Box 6.2   Potential benefits of wet wrapping

▶ Steroid use can be reduced.
▶ Reduction in or prevention of hospitalisation for the condition.
▶ Interrupts itch–scratch cycle.
▶ Cools and soothes skin.
▶ Provides mechanical barrier to scratching.
▶ Improves sleep patterns.
▶ Keeps skin hydrated.
▶ Reduces inflammation and allergy load.

---

nurse independent prescribers would treat within their competence and where they have dermatology experience they may be more likely to prescribe topical corticosteroids.

General points for prescribing in eczema include:[10]

- Hairy skin – use a lotion.
- Weeping eczema – use a cream.
- Mildly dry skin – use lotion or cream.
- Moderate, severe or widespread dry skin – use bath emollient.
- Localised flare up – short term use of topical corticosteroid (see up-to-date BNF for advice when prescribing topical corticosteroids).
- Infected flare up – take oral antibiotics.

Aim to prevent and manage flare ups by the regular use of emollients and by reviewing causative factors and avoidance where possible.

Exercise

There are several references to the evidence base for practice in this section. District Nurses commonly encounter patients with a skin problem whilst visiting for other reasons. How good is your knowledge of skin complaints? Think about the above conditions and write down the factors that would need to be taken into account prior to deciding on a form of treatment where issuing a prescription would be involved.

Palliative Care

Macmillan Gold Standards Framework

The Macmillan Gold Standards Framework[13] is a programme which promotes best practice both in primary and secondary care. It provides a framework to raise standards of palliative care by sharing resources and tools which have already been researched and practised. It was developed in order to provide equity of service in the last 6–12 months of a patient's life.[14] The patient's details are documented on a 'supportive care register' which is then monitored during a monthly meeting of the primary care team to ensure continued communication, audit and development of the palliative care service. The co-ordinator of this service in many practices is the district nurse for non-cancer palliation.

The seven aspects of care within the Gold Standards Framework include:[13]

- Communication
- Co-ordination
- Control of symptoms
- Continuity
- Continued learning
- Carer support
- Care of the dying.

Liverpool Care Pathway

The Liverpool integrated care pathway[15] has been primarily designed to assist doctors and nurses to give high quality care to patients with cancer at end of life. This approach can be adapted for use with non-cancer patients too. The tool helps to integrate national guidelines into clinical practice. It is specifically designed to be implemented in the last few days of a patient's life and supersedes other nursing care plans. Anticipatory prescribing takes place in order to promptly treat symptoms that may occur in this end stage. These recommended medicines can be prescribed by the nurse independent prescriber such as hyoscine and midazolam. Since January 2006 independent prescribers are allowed to prescribe certain controlled drugs such as diamorphine (see Appendix 1). Guidance needs to be clearer in relation to anticipatory prescribing for nurses in order to safeguard practitioners.

Preferred Place of Care[16]

As far as possible patients' views of where they would like to be looked after at the end of their life should be sought and adhered to. The Preferred Place of Care documentation is a nationally recognised tool which a patient can complete and keep to show health care professionals whenever it may be necessary to do so. For example, where an ambulance is called to take a patient to hospital, the carer or patient can show this documentation and this should prevent them being admitted when they are unable to make their wishes known. This documentation can be completed by anybody at any time during or before an illness. The proviso is that the patient is allowed to change their mind and can let health care professionals know that they wish to do so.

Prescribing in Palliative Care

Palliative care is described as the 'holistic care of patients with life-limiting diagnosis when a stage has been reached when the disease is no longer curable'.[17] Independent prescribing can be used when this stage is reached[12] and is extremely valuable in this expanding and demanding role. Many patients prefer to be cared for at home but in the past this has not always been achievable.[18] Independent prescribing can be used to help control symptoms resulting in fewer time delays while waiting for medical practitioners to visit patients or sign a prescription. Independent prescribing is also extremely beneficial to Macmillan nurses who already have a sound knowledge of the drugs prescribed in palliative care. Macmillan nurses' prescribing enhances the teamwork already promoted by the Gold Standards Framework, sharing the responsibility with the district nurses for the ultimate benefit of the patients and their carers, reducing crisis situations and avoidable hospital admissions.

Table 6.2 demonstrates some of the symptoms that are currently prescribed for in relation to palliative care and the treatments that can be prescribed where indicated.

Table 6.2 Palliative care symptoms and nurse independent prescribing drug treatment options[12,17,19,20]

Condition	Possible medication
Anxiety	Diazepam oral, parenteral, rectal Lorazepam oral, parenteral
Bowel colic	Hyoscine butylbromide parenteral
Candidiasis (oral)	Nystatin pastilles and oral suspension Miconazole oral gel and dental lacquer Fluoconazole capsules and oral solution
Confusion and restlessness	Haloperidol parenteral Midazolam parenteral Levomepromazine maleate oral Levomepromazine hydrochloride parenteral

Table 6.2 (Continued)

Condition	Possible medication
Constipation	Bulk forming laxatives Lubricants Surface wetting agents Osmotic laxatives Stimulant laxatives
Convulsions	Carbamazepine oral, rectal Gabapentin oral Midazolam parenteral
Cough	Menthol and eucalyptus inhalation Dexamethasone sodium phosphate oral Simple linctus Codeine linctus oral
Dry mouth	Artificial salivas can be prescribed
Excessive respiratory secretions	Hyoscine hydrobromide oral and parental Hyoscine butylbromide parenteral Hyoscine transdermal
Fungating malodorous tumours	Metronidazole gel external
Muscle spasm	Diazepam oral
Nausea and vomiting	Domperidone oral and rectal Levomepromazine oral and parental Metoclopramide oral and parental Cyclizine parental Haloperidol

Neuropathic pain	WHO analgesic ladder paracetamol ± NSAID
	Tricyclic antidepressants
	
	    Amitryptyline hydrochloride oral
	Anticonvulsants
	
	    Carbamazepine oral, rectal
	    Gabapentin oral
	    Imipramine hydrochloride oral

Pain control	WHO analgesic ladder
	Paracetamol preparations ±
	Ibuprofen oral, external ±
	Weak opiates
	
	    Nefopam hydrochloride oral
	    Dihydrocodeine tartrate oral
	    Codeine phosphate oral
	Strong opiates
	
	    Morphine sulphate
	    Diamorphine
	    Fentanyl (transdermal)

The NPF does not include any of the above except paracetamol and nystatin. Good symptom management is paramount in looking after patients requiring palliative care. The independent prescriber must have a sound knowledge of the drugs they prescribe, the mode of action, drug interactions and their side effects. Two common symptoms experienced by patients requiring palliative care are pain and nausea and/or vomiting. These will now be discussed in more detail

Pain

The WHO analgesic ladder shown in Figure 6.2[21] is a framework which underpins the management of pain and is used throughout the world. Initially a holistic and detailed assessment is required to establish the type of pain. A body chart and pain score is helpful when examining the cause and severity of pain.[22] An audit of pain in cancer patients[17] demonstrated that:

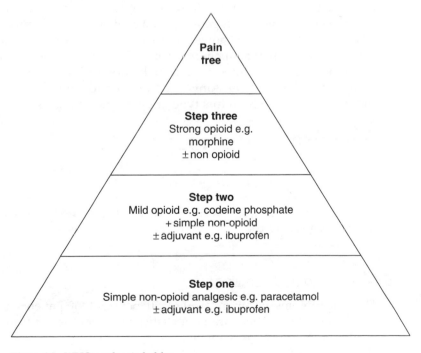

Figure 6.2 WHO analgesic ladder

▶ 33 per cent of patients have pain in one area only.
▶ 33 per cent of patients have pain in two areas.
▶ 33 per cent of patients have pain in three or more areas.

Whilst 75 per cent of patients with advanced cancer experience pain, 25 per cent do not experience any.[17] The physical, social, emotional and spiritual factors of the pain must also be considered during the assessment.[22]

In relation to independent prescribing there was a change in legislation which came into force in October 2003 to allow nurses to prescribe six controlled drugs.[23] This has been superseded by further amendments to the Home Office Misuse of Drugs Regulations from January 2006 which allow for more controlled drugs to be prescribed independently by nurse independent prescribers (see Appendix 1). Under supplementary prescribing rules, nurses can prescribe all opiates and therefore a CMP could be developed for patients requiring treatment with opioids not prescribable independently.[2]

Many patients suffer from neuropathic pain, which is caused by damage to the nervous system. The nerves may have become diseased or damaged so that they are not functioning in a normal way.[22] Neuropathic pain is generally not controlled by conventional analgesic treatments; [22,24] however, use of the analgesic ladder with non-steroidal anti inflammatory drugs (NSAIDs) as adjuvant is recommended as first-line treatment before adding other drugs such as tricyclic antidepressants or anti-epileptics which have been shown to be of benefit in this type of pain.[21] See Table 6.3.

Exercise

Palliative care has independent opportunities for the DN to assess, diagnose and treat. The medicines available are now more varied. Practitioners may lack the confidence to actually prescribe controlled drugs. How would you overcome this? What type of clinical supervision and support would you seek to confirm your competence in this area?

Nausea and Vomiting

These symptoms occur in around 50 per cent of patients with terminal cancer.[19] There are no statistics at present to confirm the incidence in non-cancer patients.

Table 6.3 Causes of nausea and vomiting in palliative care with signs and treatments

Causes of nausea and vomiting in palliative care	Signs	Treatments[12]
Treatment related	Post chemotherapy Opioid treatment	Domperidone Metoclopramide Haloperidol
Constipation	Full rectum, dyspepsia	Laxatives micro-enema
Urinary tract infection	Dysuria, frequency of micturition	Antibiotic therapy
Gastric stasis	Fullness, vomits undigested foods	Metoclopramide Levomepromazine
Hypercalcaemia	Thirst and drowsiness	Bisphosphonates
Anxiety	Worry, insomnia	Diazepam, Lorazepam, haloperidol
Cough	Vomiting post-cough	Treat cough if possible
Movement	Motion sickness	Cyclizine, haloperidol
Fungal infection	Oral candidiasis	Nystatin/Fluconazole/miconazole

The independent prescriber is able to prescribe anti-emetics but must be aware of the cause of the symptoms before any prescribing can take place.

A thorough assessment and history needs to be taken to establish the cause of the nausea and vomiting. See Table 6.3.

The detailed history should also include appetite, diet, duration of symptoms, aggravating factors, alleviating factors and the constitution of the vomit.[25] A physical examination of the mouth will be carried out to establish whether there is coating of the tongue or fungal infection of the mucosa, followed by an abdominal examination and rectal examination if appropriate to aid the diagnosis of constipation. The latter can be treated. Urine and blood tests may well also be appropriate to exclude urinary tract infection and hypercalcaemia, which may also present with thirst and drowsiness.[17] At all times the independent prescriber should contribute to correcting the reversible cause and by using a holistic approach try non-drug methods first. It may be as simple as avoiding the smell of cooking food that may be the trigger or practising some relaxation techniques.[25]

Drug treatment may be necessary. The initial treatment for gastric stasis where there is no intestinal obstruction, perforation or haemorrhage is normally metoclopramide.[19] Domperidone is used in nausea and vomiting caused by cytotoxic therapy and is beneficial because it is less sedating than other anti-emetics. Both of these drugs are dopamine-receptor antagonists. They antagonise dopamine receptors in the chemoreceptor zone located in the postrema of the brain. They also aid gastric emptying.[1] Cyclizine is used for motion sickness, raised intracranial pressure and organic bowel obstruction.[1] Cyclizine is an antihistamine which works on the vomiting centre of the brain inhibiting the action of the histamine. Levomepromazine is a second-line anti-emetic which blocks the chemoreceptor trigger zone.

District nurses would ensure that the treatment they have prescribed is effective by closely monitoring the patient's symptoms as they would be visiting them on a regular basis.

An anti-emetic such as haloperidol may be the treatment of choice. It has similar characteristics to that of levomepromazine but is used for chemical causes of vomiting and is generally non-sedating as well as being a useful anti-psychotic if the patient is suffering from hallucinations associated with strong opioid treatments.

Supplementary Prescribing

Supplementary prescribing is an option available when prescribing. The supplementary prescriber is able to prescribe anything in the BNF including controlled, unlicensed and off-license medicines.[2] See Chapter 3 for a definition of supplementary prescribing.

Patients on the district nursing caseload who are housebound with conditions such as newly diagnosed hypertension may benefit from the district nurse being an independent or supplementary prescriber if this falls within her/his competence. The district nurse would give advice such as dietary, exercise and lifestyle health in the first instance as lifestyle risk reduction can result in blood pressure lowering.[26] Prior to commencing drug treatment other risk factors such as diabetes and previous myocardial infarction will be taken into account as well as a cardiovascular disease risk (CVD) prediction, which includes the risk of stroke.[27] CVD prediction charts can be found at the back of the BNF from No. 49,

March 2005.[12] Prior to this the charts in the BNF were only available for coronary risk prediction. The district nurse would be responsible for monitoring the patient's blood pressure and it makes sense for her/him to titrate medication and add in new medication where required following national and local guidelines. An example of a CMP for hypertension based on national guidance can be found in Appendix 2. All CMPs must be patient specific and therefore it is important when using a template to ensure that it is adapted to reflect the patient's medical and medicines history. For instance ACE inhibitors would be contraindicated in patients with renal artery stenosis. The National Institute for Clinical Excellence (NICE)[28,29] and the British Hypertension Society (BHS)[27] differ in their advice for treatment thresholds and target blood pressures. These are shown in Table 6.4.

Table 6.4 Hypertension treatment thresholds and target blood pressures[30]

	NICE 2002 and 2004[28,29]	BHS 2004[27]
Blood pressure treatment initiating thresholds mmHg		
Without diabetes	>140/90 (NICE) >140–159/90 (BHS)	If 10-year CVD risk ≥20 per cent or existing CVD or Target Organ Damage
	≥160/ ≥100 NICE and BHS	Treat all patients
With diabetes	≥140/80 (NICE) ≥140/90 (BHS)	Treat if 10-year CVD risk >20 per cent or history of CVD or concomitant microalbuminuria or proteinuria	Treat all patients
	≥160/≥100 (NICE and BHS)	Treat all patients
Target BP mmHg Systolic+diastolic (S+D)		
Without diabetes S+D	≤140/90	<14085
With diabetes S+D	<140/80 or ≤135/75 if microalbuminuria or proteinuria present	<130/80

Source: Adapted from National Prescribing Centre (Unpublished presentation).

Other conditions which might be appropriate to non-medical prescribing for district nurses include: Type 2 diabetes mellitus; hypothyroidism and palliative care (as mentioned previously in this chapter). In practice it is more difficult to implement supplementary prescribing where there is no immediate access to a patient's medical records but by following safeguards such as obtaining relevant new information prior to visiting a patient at home it can be achieved quite successfully.

Exercise

Consider a disease area with which you are familiar. Consider the symptoms and complications associated with this disease/illness. Write a list of medicines commonly used in treatment. Find the evidence for this. Look up the dosage, indications, contraindications, interactions, side effects and pharmacology of at least three of these.

Conclusion

Prescribing is already in the remit of qualified district nurses, and independent and supplementary prescribing could become an invaluable part of a district nurse's toolkit. Whilst the NPF may be useful for basic nursing practice, the changes to the role of the qualified district nurse must include the wider prescribing remit.

The current NPF may be far too limited for any district nursing sister to work from as it is unlikely to meet the demands of the role. Wider prescribing is more in keeping with the role of district nurses and their teams in the twenty-first century, particularly in relation to the areas covered in this chapter. Patients can only benefit from district nursing teams being willing to embrace these enhanced roles as they are often the main health care contact for patients who are housebound. They are often the ones to diagnose minor illnesses in these patients. The district nursing role in palliative care is well recognised and being able to prescribe in this area prevents unnecessary delays and further suffering for patients who are at the end stage of their lives.

References

1. Courtenay, M. and Butler, M. *Essential Nurse Prescribing* (London: GMM, 2002).

2. DH. *Supplementary Prescribing by Nurses, Pharmacists, Chiropodists/Podiatrists, Physiotherapists and Radiographers within the NHS in England* (London: DH, 2005).

3. Brookes, D. 'Community assessment of diabetic foot ulcers'. *Journal of Community Nursing*, 15: 2 (2001) 34–38.

4. Addison, D., Rennison, T. and Del Bono, M. 'The antimicrobial properties of a silver alginate dressing for moderate to heavily exuding wounds'. *Journal of Wound, Ostomy & Continence Nursing*, 32: 3 (2005) Supplement 2.

5. Brookes, D. 'Selecting and developing independent and supplementary nurse prescribers'. *Nurse Prescribing*, 2: 5 (2004) 212–216.

6. NMC. *Code of Professional Conduct* (London: NMC, 2004).

7. Basford, L. 'Maintaining nurse prescribing competence: Experiences and challenges'. *Nurse Prescribing*, 1: 1 (2003) 40–45.

8. Graham-Brown, R. and Bourke, J. *Mosby's Color Atlas and Text of Dermatology* (London: Mosby, 1998).

9. Page, B. 'The benefits of tubifast garments in the management of atopic eczema'. *British Journal of Nursing*, 14: 5 (2005) 289–291.

10. Prodigy. *Prodigy guidance: Atopic eczema.* 2nd edition (London: The Stationary Office, 2005).

11. Skin Care World. *Wet Wrapping Efficacy.* www.skincareworld.co.uk accessed 24 June 2005.

12. BMA/RPSGB. *British National Formulary.* No. 49 (London: BMA/RPSGB, March 2005).

13. Macmillan. *Gold Standards Framework.* www.goldstandardsframework.nhs.uk accessed 30 May 2005.

14. Collins, F. 'Using gold standards to raise awareness of palliative care'. *Nursing Times*, 100: 48 (30 November 2004) 30–31.

15. LCP. Liverpool Care Pathway. www.lcp-mariecurie.org.uk, accessed 13 July 2005.

16. Cancer Lancashire. Preferred Place of Care. www.cancerlancashire.org.uk/ppchtml, accessed 20 February 2006.

17. Twycross, R. *Introducing Palliative Care*. 4th Edition (Oxford: Radcliffe Medical Press, 2003) p. 2.

18. Pemberton, C. *Speaking of dying . . .* Edline Royal College of Nursing, Autumn 2004.

19. Kaye, P. *A–Z Pocketbook of Symptom Control* (Northampton: EPL Publications, 1998).

20. Faull, C. and Woof, R. *Palliative Care* (Oxford: Oxford University Press, 2002).

21. World Health Organisation (WHO). *Cancer Pain Relief* (Geneva: WHO, 1996).

22. Bamkin, D. 'Nurse prescribing in a palliative care setting: Brachial plexus pain'. *Nurse Prescribing*, 2: 4 (2004) 174–176.

23. HMSO. Statutory Instrument 2003 No. 2429. The Misuse of Drugs (Amendment) (No.3) Regulations 2003 (London: HMSO, 2003).

24. McGann, C. 'Treating chronic pain: The nurse's role and the impact of supplementary prescribing'. *Nurse Prescribing*, 1: 3 (2003) 120–126.

25. Close, H. 'Nausea and vomiting in terminally ill patients: Towards a holistic approach'. *Nurse Prescribing*, 1: 1 (2003) 22–26.

26. Geleijnse, J., Kok, F. and Grobbee, D. 'Impact of Dietary and Lifestyle Factors on the prevalence of hypertension in Western Populations'. *European Journal of Public Health*, 14 (2004) 235–239.

27. Williams, B., Poulter, N., Brown, M., Davis, M., McInnes, G., Potter, J., Sever, P. and McGThom, S. 'Guidelines for management of hypertension: Report of the fourth working party of the British Hypertension Society'. *Journal of Human Hypertension*, 18 (2004) 139–185.

28. NICE. *Hypertension Guidelines* (London: NICE, 2002).

29. NICE. *Hypertension – Management of Hypertension in Adults in Primary Care* (London: NICE, 2004).

30. NPC. *Management of Hypertension.* Unpublished Seminar (2005).

Useful website

End of Life NHS Site   www.endoflife.nhs.uk

Chapter 7

Midwifery perspectives

Jenny Prior

Introduction

This chapter will consider the need for midwives to prescribe medicines for women in their care. There exist various legislative Acts, subsequent amendments to these Acts and statutory instruments (SIs) (shown in Box 7.1) which provide midwives with the ability to 'supply and administer' medicines often used in maternity care provision without the need for a prescription or a PGD. The legislation for the supply and administration of POMs consists of exemptions for midwives in the Acts and SIs.

Box 7.1 Legislation relating to supply and administration of medicines by midwives

Medicines Act 1968 (as amended)
Misuse of Drugs Act 1971 (as amended)

Various SIs amending the Medicines Act:

Pharmacy (P) and General Sales List (GSL) medicines, SI 1980 Order No. 1924, The Medicines (P and GSL exemption) Order 1980.
Prescription Only Medicines (POMs), SI 1997 Order No. 1830, The Prescription Only Medicines (human Use) Order 1997.
Misuse of Drugs, SI 2001, Order No. 3998, Misuse of Drugs Regulations 2001 (amendment to the 1971 Misuse of Drugs Act).

Table 7.1 POMs that can be supplied and/or administered by midwives

Midwives may supply only	Midwives may administer only
Chloral hydrate	Diamorphine
Ergometrine malleate (only	Ergometrine malleate
when contained in a	Lignocaine (Lidocaine) (in labour only)
medicinal product which	Lignocaine hydrochloride (Lidocaine
is *not* for parenteral	hydrochloride) (in labour only)
administration)	Morphine
Pentazocine hydrochloride	Naloxone hydrochloride
Phytomenadione	Oxytocins (natural and synthetic)
Triclofos sodium	Pentazocine hydrochloride
	Pethidine hydrochloride
	Phytomenadione
	Promazine hydrochloride (in labour only)

Table 7.1 shows the list of medicines that midwives can supply and/or administer without the need for a prescription or PGD in the course of their professional practice. They appear in the Prescription Only Medicines (Human Use) Order 1997.[1] This also includes diamorphine and morphine for administration purposes, which were added to the amended 1997 Order in 2004.[2]

In addition to these medicines, the Midwives Rules and Standards[3] state that:

> You are able to supply and administer all non-prescription medicines which include all pharmacy and general sales list medicines without a prescription. (Rule 7, p. 19)

Therefore, midwives are able to supply and administer a variety of medicines without a prescription or PGD and from the Pharmacy (P) and General Sales List (GSL) medicines. The Midwives Rules and Standards also state that:

> a practising midwife shall only supply and administer those medicines, including analgesics, in respect of which she has received the appropriate training as to use, dosage and methods of administration.[3]

Interpretation of the Law

As can be seen from above the law in this area is rather complicated and can be open to misinterpretation. Confusion also exists regarding the understanding of the terms 'prescribing', POM, P,

GSL, 'standing orders' and PGDs. Midwives are the lead professionals in normal maternity care provision.[4] Due to the physiological changes in pregnancy, some women may experience a number of ailments that may require medicinal treatment. Generally speaking, women should be advised to take as little as possible in the way of medicines during pregnancy, labour and puerperal period. However, on occasions it may be necessary when the benefit outweighs any risk, to the mother, fetus and/or the breastfeeding neonate to prescribe, supply or administer medication. Examples of conditions that may require treatment include:

- headaches
- heartburn (may be due to relaxation of the cardiac sphincter)
- vulvovaginal candidiasis (thrush), which may be due to a change in pH of the vagina in pregnancy.

Medicines to alleviate and treat these conditions can be legally supplied and administered by the midwife without the need for a prescription. Midwives in the hospital may receive stock from the hospital pharmacy. Community midwives previously carried medicines to treat these conditions or accessed them from their local dispensing GP practice where they would have been based. However, following violence against midwives and not being based at the GP practice, this has all but ceased in the community setting. In these circumstances it would be of benefit to midwives if they could prescribe such medicines.

Midwives may find non-medical prescribing a helpful tool. This may be ideal for those working in specialisms such as diabetes, drugs liaison or 'Surestart' where they may be involved in family planning services. There are opportunities in the family planning arena for midwives to prescribe as generally the women are well and will not need referral to a doctor unless there are underlying or other medical conditions. For those working with homeless women, travelling communities, refugees and asylum seekers, prescribing may benefit women, enhancing midwives' autonomy.

Independent Prescribing for Midwives

Identifiable health care professionals, including midwives, can undertake a degree or postgraduate level prescribing course in order for them to become non-medical prescribers. It is recommended that the midwife should have at least 3 years of post-registration experience prior to undertaking the course (see Chapter 2). On qualifying, midwives can prescribe from the BNF for conditions falling within their competence. The BNF includes appendices highlighting medicines that may be prescribed to women during pregnancy and while breastfeeding, and includes those that might put the fetus or baby at risk. These appendices are a very useful inclusion for midwives and helps them in the decision-making processes.

Supplementary Prescribing for Midwives

Supplementary prescribing was introduced in 2003,[5] to ease pressures on doctors' time and to improve access of the general public to medicines.[6] There are differences in how supplementary prescribing works in comparison to independent prescribing. Midwives prescribing in a supplementary role must work jointly with the independent prescriber (a doctor), review patients at regular, pre-arranged intervals and implement a specific CMP. Once the midwife, doctor and the woman have agreed on this plan, the midwife may prescribe any medicine that appears on the plan until it is reviewed jointly by all parties. There are no restrictions on the medical conditions that can be managed by the supplementary prescriber, except that the midwife must only prescribe within her/his competence.

As from April 2005 supplementary prescribing was extended to include controlled drugs and unlicensed medicines under the amendments to the Misuse of Drugs Regulations 2001.[7]

Standing Orders

Local policies referred to as 'standing orders' were partly devised due to the impracticality of individual midwives carrying their own supply of medicines. They have also been used to supplement the legislation according to the NMC.[3] The term does not exist in the medicines legislation. The NMC also state that they do not need to be replaced by PGDs (p. 20).[3]

PGDs

The PGDs allow many POMs, P and GSL medicines to be supplied and/or administered to patients under specific circumstances[8] (see Chapter 18). PGDs came about as the result of a report on the supply and administration of medicines, the legal framework for PGDs being put in place in 2000[9] and 2001 in Northern Ireland.[10] PGDs need to be signed by a doctor (usually an obstetrician for maternity use) and pharmacist. Midwives who will be working under the PGD must sign to say they have been educated in its use and that they agree to work within its confines. The senior midwife may be a signatory at its inception.

In October 2003 the Misuse of Drugs Regulations 2001 were amended to allow some controlled drugs to be supplied and administered under a PGD.[11] Consequently there are copious PGDs in Acute NHS Trusts with these added. This is not necessary for midwives as they can already supply and administer those controlled drugs used in maternity care as part of the 1968 Medicines Act exemptions and the amended 1971 Misuse of Drugs Act.[12,13]

It is important that PGDs do not replace prescribing on an individual basis as this is the safest mode for the majority of women in maternity care to receive medicines. Therefore PGDs should not cover long-term conditions such as diabetes or asthma. Supplementary prescribing, however, would be ideal for treating women with long-term conditions where the specialist midwife is working jointly alongside the doctor.

Prescribing and Midwifery

For health and safety reasons, Acute NHS Trusts and Primary Care Trusts have set parameters in relation to the number of occasions that a medicine can be administered by midwives. For example, in some Trusts paracetamol or gaviscon may only be given on two occasions. This is to ensure that conditions such as pregnancy-induced hypertension (PIH) or pre-eclampsia, which can present with symptoms of headaches and epigastric pain, are not missed by the midwife. In the community, a woman may be advised to take paracetamol from her own supply or it could be supplied by the midwife. In theory, in the primary care setting, the woman could take more than two consecutive doses to control a headache.

The midwife would have given instructions to contact herself or a doctor if there was no significant improvement after a certain time period had elapsed. As an independent prescriber the midwife has more autonomy and can use her professional judgement as she is able to *prescribe* for such conditions rather than *administer* only.

A woman may need more than two doses of paracetamol for other reasons, for example for perineal pain or for 'after pains' following childbirth. This is where once again independent prescribing would be a valuable asset for midwives. It could be argued that where there is a lack of independent prescribers, a delay potentially causing pain and morbidity to women might occur.

When a medicine is being provided to a woman for the first time, under a PGD, the midwife will record the name of the drug, time given and dosage on the appropriate drug chart (sometimes called a 'prescription chart'). This is not 'prescribing' in the true, legal sense of the word; it is merely entering the information required onto the drug chart for the safe administration of medicine at that time and on subsequent occasions. It is not necessary either for the midwife to find a prescriber to sign the prescription chart in these circumstances. However, midwives working in the role of a prescriber may use the hospital drug/prescription charts to prescribe medicines from the formulary for other midwives to supply and administer. In the community setting, independent prescribers can issue a prescription.

Supply of Medicines

In hospital, medicines are readily supplied to the wards and labour suites by hospital pharmacy. The medicines are stored appropriately. In the community setting there are several issues to consider:

▶ Where does the midwife obtain her supply?
▶ How is it obtained?
▶ Where can the medicines be stored?

In order to obtain supplies the supervisor of midwives must complete and sign a supply order stating the midwife's name and occupation. It must also contain the purpose for which the drug is required and the total quantity to be obtained. The medicines must then be stored according to the legislation. This can be a problem where midwives are not working at a base with adequate storage facilities. Controlled and other drugs used to be supplied by a pharmacist to a community midwife for use in childbirth using a supply order signed by the supervisor of midwives or medical officer. If a controlled drug had been obtained from a pharmacy by a supply order, the midwife could return the opiate to them if it was unused. However, few drugs are now carried (with the exception of ergometrine maleate with oxytocin). Currently if a woman requires controlled drugs to be available for her confinement, they are her legal responsibility. In this instance because the prescription is for the named person, unused medicines cannot be returned to a pharmacy by the midwife. The woman herself may return it to the pharmacy from where it was obtained. Alternatively, the woman can be encouraged to destroy it herself, ideally in the presence of the midwife.[3]

Conclusion

Some midwives may feel that they have sufficient scope under existing legislation relating to the supply and administration of medicines. However, there is an argument for the benefits of becoming independent and supplementary prescribers, as this would enhance the care, particularly for those women requiring the attentions of specialist midwives. It may also give them more autonomy and job satisfaction.

References

1. DH. *Prescription Only Medicines (Human Use) Order* (London: DH, 1997). www.hmso.gov.uk, accessed 12/04/05.

2. NMC. *Addition of Diamorphine and Morphine to the List of Exemptions of Medicines for Midwives. The Prescription Only Medicines (Human Use) Amendment Order 2004.* Circular 10/2004/27 (London: NMC, April 2004).

3. NMC. *Midwives Rules and Standards* (London: NMC, 2004).

4. NICE. *Antenatal Care: Routine Care for the Healthy Pregnant Woman* (London: NICE, 2003).

5. DH. *Supplementary Prescribing by Nurses and Pharmacologists within the NHS in England* (London: DH, 2003).

6. Modernisation Agency. *Medicine Matters: A Guide to Current Mechanisms for the Prescribing, Supply and Administration of Medicines. MDA, Changing Workforce Programme, DH Care Prescribing Group* (London: DH, 2005).

7. DH. *Summary of Changes to Regulations on Supplementary Prescribing and Guidelines/Medicines Pharmacy and Industry/Prescriptions* (London: DH, 2005). www.dh.gov.uk/policy, accessed 12/04/05.

8. DH. *Patient Group Directions (England only)*. HSC 2000/026 (London: DH, 2000).

9. NPC. *Framework for Patient Group Directions*. NPC, NHS. www.npc.co.uk; www.npc.nhs.uk, accessed 12/04/05 (2004).

10. DHSSPS. *Guidance: Patient Group Directions* (Northern Ireland: DHSSPS, 2001).

11. DH. *Misuse of Drug Regulations* (London: DH, 2001).

12. DH. *Misuse of Drugs Act* (London: DH, 1971).

13. NMC. *Medicines Legislation: What it Means for Midwives*. Circular 1/2005, 06/01/05 (London: NMC, 2005).

Chapter 8

Health visitor perspectives

Jill Davies

Introduction

Health visiting has always had its foundations in public health, but changing priorities have brought about challenges.[1] Policy documents throughout the United Kingdom identified areas for priority action with regard to inequalities in health, an increasing ageing population and premature deaths from such diseases as cancer and coronary heart disease. Alongside these targets for practice came the emergence of non-medical prescribing, which further challenged health visitors to identify their expertise. This chapter will discuss the public health role of the health visitor and how prescribing may fit in with the wider health visiting agenda.

Background

Recent policy documents have highlighted the changing face of health visiting, including Liberating the Talents,[2] which identified new family-centred public health roles for health visitors. These new roles aim to strengthen the community-based public health role, focusing on individuals, families and community working. The Health Visitor and School Nurse Development Programme[3] presents a comprehensive agenda for health visitors concerning their expertise and the inter-agency working ethos. Whilst this is not a dynamic change, it does provide health visitors with flexibility of working and enables a more integrated approach focussing on improving client care and working across traditional boundaries.

An integral aspect of the specialist practitioner programme for health visitor training is successful completion of a course of study that enables them to prescribe from the NPF. This formulary comprises a number of medicines (POM and GSL medicines) along with dressings, creams and appliances relevant to community nursing and health visiting.

It is now recognised that having the skills and qualification to prescribe from the NPF is part of a health visitor's role. Following on from the initial pilot studies[4,5] and successful evaluation, nurse prescribing was rolled out across the country to all health care professionals who had either a health visitor or district nurse qualification. More recent studies have suggested that health visitors may not be utilising this added skill. Rodden[6] highlighted in a survey of 32 health visitors that 70 per cent were writing less than five prescriptions a week. While and Biggs[7] found that health visitors were generally prescribing for conditions such as lice infestations, skin conditions (dry skin, dermatitis) and medicines for oral fungal infections. The limitations to the NPF may be preventing a wider application of the prescribing role.

Health Visiting

As previously stated, the role of the health visitor has its roots in public health and health promotion. It is historically focused on the needs of families and children. The initial contact with clients usually commences during the postnatal period.[8] Health visitors' roles have evolved following policy directives such as the formation of the third part of the NMC register which focuses on public health. They are unique in being one of the few professionals who visit the well population, with the intention of promoting health. They can be working with diverse client groups including home visits to parents with young children, community groups and travellers. For some health visitors the role involves supporting people from the cradle to grave. It includes working in areas such as accident prevention, teenage parenting, substance misuse, homelessness, domestic violence, child protection and mental health.[2] Some health visitors provide a service to an elderly population, for example 'over 75' screening. Smith[9] identified that health visitors referred to their 'practice' as family centred, delivering health promotion programmes to individuals and families, these being mainly mothers and preschool children. This study also highlighted that the public health role is constrained by the need to be reactive to caseload practice.

Exercise

Health visitors are now being trained as Specialist Community Public Health Nurses. How will their prescribing remit complement the role?

Health visitors are adopting new and dynamic roles. Does the Community practitioner's Formulary offer sufficient scope? What difference would it make if they could prescribe from the full formulary?

Prescribing

Although, as previously identified, prescribing is an aspect of health visiting practice, it is interesting to note that there is no reference to prescribing in the defining document 'The Health Visitor and School Nurse Development Programme'.[3] There is a general lack of evidence for the benefits of health visitor prescribing. This could suggest that prescribing is not seen to be a part of the health visitor role; on the other hand it could be argued that it has already become such a part of the role that people are no longer looking for evidence to support the practice.

Health visitors were one of the first professional groups identified to develop prescribing within their role and it is somewhat surprising that they have not truly embraced this.[10]

It was suggested at a Royal College of Nursing International Research Conference in 2004 that health visitors were often refusing to take their prescription pads with them on visits as they were perceiving that prescribing was more trouble than it was worth.[10] Prescribing may be problematic as the action needs to be documented in health records in a GP surgery.[10] This could result in a health visitor returning to a GP practice to complete the record keeping, which has significant implications on their time. They could, however, come to an arrangement with the GP surgeries to fax or telephone prescriptions through confidential systems as these communication tools are already in place for other health professionals such as out-of-hours services.

Following the preliminary pilot studies,[4,5] prescribing for health visitors became mandatory. This was a specific issue as many of them felt that this had been a compulsory change in their role, without consultation. The apparent reluctance from some health visitors to prescribe may reflect this feeling. There may be other reasons for the lack of enthusiasm and some argue that health visitors do not have the pharmacological knowledge to prescribe.[11] This may support the argument for those who do not see prescribing as part of their public health role. Others, however, may feel that they are in a prime position to prescribe as part of that role, for instance by providing smoking cessation services or family planning advice. It would make sense for them to be able to complete the episode of care by offering a prescription following appropriate advice.

One area of management identified by Groat[12] is that of prescribing for the treatment of eczema in children as there is more scope for treatment as an independent prescriber, Davies, concurs.[10] Topical corticosteroids which are an appropriate treatment in the management of inflamed eczema may be prescribed (see Chapter 6).

Conclusion

Various documents have been published which give direction for developing health visiting practice[13] although it is worth noting that these do not explicitly state that prescribing is part of the role.

Extending prescribing rights for health visitors could be seen as an essential tool to enable progress by improving access to medication and increasing clients' choice, as advocated by the first Crown Report.[14] It will take the skills of a well-informed health visitor to work creatively on uniting these policies with the added skills of the full prescribing formulary as many have rejected the NPF.[15] Whilst some health visitors will not see this as an advantage within the public health arena, others may feel just the opposite.

The discussion within this chapter highlights the diverse role of the health visitor. What may be appropriate for one may be very different for another. Whether one supports the view that health visitors should become nurse independent prescribers or not, history has shown that the training should remain optional, as research suggests that compulsory training has not been effective in this area of practice.

References

1. Department of Health. *The NHS Plan* (London: DH, 2000).

2. Department of Health. *Liberating the Talents: Helping Primary Care Trusts and Nurses to Deliver the NHS Plan* (London: DH, 2002).

3. Department of Health. *Health Visitor and School Nurse Development Programme* (London: DH, 2001).

4. Luker, K., Austin, L., Hogg, C. and Willock, J. *Evaluation of Nurse Prescribing Final Report* (The University of Liverpool and The University of York, 1997).

5. Luker, K., Austin, L., Hogg, C., Ferguson, B. and Smith, K. 'Nurse-patient relationships: The context of nurse prescribing'. *Journal of Advanced Nursing*, 28: 2 (1998) 235–242.

6. Rodden, C. 'Nurse prescribing: Views on autonomy and independence'. *British Journal of Community Nursing*, 6: 7 (2001) 350–355.

7. While, A. and Biggs, K. 'Benefits and challengers of nurse prescribing'. *Journal of Advanced Nursing*, 45: 6 (2004) 559–567.

8. Cody, A. 'Health visiting as a therapy'. *Journal of Advanced Nursing*, 29: 1 (1999) 119–127.

9. Smith, M.A. 'Health visiting: The public health role'. *Journal of Advanced Nursing*, 45: 1 (2004) 17–25.

10. Davies, J. (2005) 'Health Visitors Perceptions of Nurse Prescribing', accepted for publication Nurse Prescriber.

11. Whiles, A. and Rees, K. 'Health visitors' knowledge of products to be included in the nurses' formulary'. *Health Visitor*, 67: 2 (1994) 57–58.

12. Groat, D. 'Eczema care for children: The health visitor's role expanded'. *Community Practitioner*, 75: 2 (2002) 54–56.

13. Hall, S. *Health for All Children*. 4th edition (Oxford: Oxford Medical, 2003).

14. Department of Health. *Report of the Advisory Group on Nurse Prescribing Crown 1* (London: HMSO, 1989).

15. McCaughan, D. 'Health visitors reject prescribing as too limited'. *Nursing Standard*, 18: 29 (2004) 8.

Chapter 9

Mental health nursing perspectives

Simon Sherring and Adrian Rendall

Introduction

The advent of independent and supplementary prescribing for nurses is an exciting development within mental health care, with dramatic implications for patient care and mental health nursing as a profession. There has been much debate regarding mental health nurses' prescribing. The profession is cautiously welcoming this change. In embracing it, the nurses need to ensure these changes are delivered in a manner that is helpful to service users, and seen as an expansion of the role of the mental health nurse, rather than a means of meeting service shortfalls. This chapter will discuss some of the issues surrounding this practice within the clinical setting and how the role might enhance the service offered to clients.

Exploring Prescribing Potential

Many busy nurses welcome the convenience of writing a prescription, for example, to intervene early at a time of crisis, thus enabling the service user to obtain speedy access to medication. Some people may argue that when providing advice and guidance to GPs and Senior House Officers that nurses have been prescribing indirectly. However, nurse prescribing is more than legitimising de-facto prescribing, it is about capitalising on the existing skills, experience and knowledge mental health nurses have in caring for service users. Research from the United States regarding prescribing has shown no difference in outcomes for service users between nurse prescribers and medical practitioners,[1] but nurse prescribing has been associated with:

▶ improved service user education
▶ increased recognition of side effects
▶ greater continuity of care
▶ improved adherence with medication plans.[2]

The experience of mental health nurses in the United States also suggests that nurse prescribing can lead to a reduction in waiting times to see psychiatrists, and an increase in the quality of care with greater service user satisfaction.[2] It is anticipated that similar benefits would be felt by mental health nurses and service users in the United Kingdom. It is encouraging that small-scale studies suggest that service users are happy with nurse prescribers[3,4] and that prescribing could be provided at considerably lower cost than that of physicians, with the potential for equivalent or better outcomes.[5]

The role of the nurse in medicines management now has greater potential than ever before. There is still a role for supplementary prescribing in mental health as the prescribing decisions work through partnerships with medical practitioners and service users. There is some concern that supplementary prescribing may potentially compromise nurses, since some psychiatrists fail to comply with prescribing guidelines.[6] Essentially this could result in unacceptable levels of polypharmacy, inappropriate high doses of medication and an underutilisation of new treatments. Nurses must ensure that they protect service users from poor prescribing; ensuring that prescriptions are evidence based and follow national guidance, for example NICE Guidelines. Whilst independent prescribing allows nurses to prescribe and alter medication according to the evidence base, some still lack confidence in their competence. Supplementary prescribing, however, in spite of concerns, provides an opportunity for nurses to contribute to improvements in medication treatment plans, and confront poor prescribing practice as CMPs refer to appropriate guidelines for practice.

Exercise

It can be difficult to act assertively towards medical colleagues when advocating for a client. Are you able to be assertive when the necessity arises? Ask a colleague to enact a role play in which both of you consider your opinions about a treatment are correct. Ask another colleague to observe the interaction and report on your behaviour

Setting the Trend

Of the 44 Trusts in England, surveyed by the Institute of Psychiatry in 2004, 102 mental health nurses had completed training in independent and supplementary prescribing. A further 128 mental health nurses were undertaking the training.[1] Although these figures are relatively low, it is anticipated that prescribing will become a rapid area of development for nurses and other health care professionals, particularly in community-based services.[1] It is apparent that some areas in the United Kingdom have embraced nurse prescribing more enthusiastically than others. The pace of growth is faster in England at present. Other parts of the United Kingdom would benefit greatly from mental health nurse prescribing as current policy ensures that funding is focused in the areas poorly served by medical staff. This applies to those in remote rural areas and inner city areas, where it is difficult to recruit psychiatrists. Many nurses have experience of taking additional training to deliver specialist interventions, such as family work for schizophrenia and cognitive behavioural interventions, which would enhance their prescribing role. Nurses should ensure that prescribing takes place within a broad range of interventions when making changes to treatment plans, thus enhancing partnership within the prescribing relationship. To prevent nurses feeling overwhelmed with change and to capitalise on this experience, adequate resources, planning and support will need to be given (see Chapter 19).

Optimising Treatment

Nurses working in mental health care are well placed to take advantage of the narrow window of opportunity when a service user contemplates accepting medication or changing a prescription. Medication management is a core-nursing role, which sets apart mental health nurses from other members of the multi-disciplinary team in relation to this area of practice.[7] Independent and supplementary prescribing represents an opportunity for them to add to their skills in medicines management and avoid some of the potential pitfalls that may be encountered.

Case study

A 24-year-old gentleman suffers from schizophrenia. He is under the care of an Assertive Outreach Team as he is unable to keep regular appointments with mental health services. He lives alone and has little social contact. It is very difficult to arrange a medical review as he does not attend the outpatients department; because he was admitted to hospital the last time he went there. Medical reviews have been arranged at his home address; however, he is frequently not at home for the appointment. He has not seen his general practitioner in many years. The members of the Assertive Outreach Team maintain intermittent contact with him by repeatedly visiting his home address in the hope that he will be there, and visiting places that he frequents, for example a local cafe. The Team review his treatment when they see him. When they do see him, he is not always very talkative. On occasions he does speak to the team members, and this allows them to make an assessment of his mental state. Traditionally if there are changes in his mental state they would have to be reported back to the consultant psychiatrist for changes to be made to his medication. This might take some time, and mean a delay in changing medication or starting new medication. This would be further complicated by having to try to meet the man again. It is during this narrow window of opportunity that a nurse prescriber could have a positive impact on his mental state. A nurse independent prescriber could prescribe medications as required. If the nurse lacks confidence they could alter doses or add medicines through a supplementary prescribing partnership within a pre-agreed CMP, for example increasing the dose of antipsychotic medication. See for example Clinical Management Plan in Appendix 2.

Training Requirements

Few nurses, in the authors' experience, would dispute the suggestion that mental health nurses' knowledge of psychopharmacology and the biological basis of mental illness is weak.[7] In this context, it is clear that there needs to be a creative, flexible and comprehensive curriculum for their preparation to competently fulfil the role of prescriber. The relationships with the consultant psychiatrist and pharmacist are likely to be a key element to the success of non-medical prescribing. Practitioners wishing to undertake training are required to have a medical practitioner as a mentor/assessor. It is anticipated that psychiatrists will see the training of nurse prescribers as an opportunity to free them to address more complicated psychopathology; however, time would need to be set aside for them to provide nurse prescribers with adequate support.

Service Improvements

With the need to contain cost, increase access to quality mental health care and improve service user satisfaction, it is easy to see why the government have extended prescribing authority to nurses. Although nurse prescribing remains contentious to some,[8] there are clearly a number of potential benefits.

These benefits may include mental health services being more responsive to service user needs. For example:

▶ intervening early
▶ more effective management of side effects
▶ considerate and responsive titration of medication doses.

As previously mentioned, there is often a narrow window of opportunity when service users with long-term mental health conditions are prepared to consider medication. These service users might include those in crisis or those with difficulty in engagement. Nurses are well placed to take advantage of these opportunities. Mental health nurses can provide portable prescribing, meeting the needs of service users in their own surroundings and on their own terms. This flexibility may include the time of contact or the location.

There may be positive changes in service user's experiences of mental health care, for example by sharing the responsibility of care with them and helping them to manage their medications more effectively. Nurse prescribing may lead to improvements in engagement, concordance and outcomes if delivered within a positive therapeutic alliance with service users.

Supplementary prescribing offers opportunities for secondary care nurses, to be more flexible in the way they practice and embrace policy initiatives.[9] With appropriate use of independent and supplementary prescribing, nurses can take a lead in arranging rapid admissions and discharges from hospital, relieving the pressure on beds and making services more user-centred.[10,11] Many nurses will have had the frustrating experience of managing service users who no longer require this environment and are keen to be discharged, however, remain on the acute wards for days, waiting to be reviewed by a psychiatrist at a ward round. With the impact of European Working Time Directives and Modernising Medical Careers, psychiatrists could spend more time at a ward round with service users who are acutely unwell.[12]

Conclusion

In conclusion, non-medical prescribing represents an exciting opportunity for mental health nurses to improve patient care. However, it is a momentous practice change that requires sensitive, cautious and effective change management. There are a number of exciting challenges to be overcome in maximising the success of its implementation. There may be some service users who do not wish to accept the role of the nurse prescriber, and this would need to be respected. The success of nurse prescribing will depend heavily on the relationships established between the service user, and the nurses who must be adequately prepared to embrace the change. The organisation's role is pivotal in ensuring that the appropriate infrastructure is in place to prepare and support prescribers.

References

1. National Prescribing Centre, the National Institute for Mental Health in England and the Department of Health. *Improving Mental Health Services by Extending the Role of Nurses in Prescribing and Supplying Medication: Good Practice Guide* (London: DH, 2005).

2. Nolan, P. 'Mental health nurses perceptions of nurse prescribing'. *The Journal of Advanced Nursing*, 36: 4 (2001) 527–534.

3. Aldridge, S. 'Nurse practitioners are hit with patients'. *British Medical Journal*, 324 (2002) 819–823.

4. Brooks, N., Otway, C. and Rashid, C. 'The patient's view: The benefits and limits of nurse prescribing'. *British Journal of Community Nursing*, 6: 7 (2001) 342–348.

5. Bardell, J. 'Clinical outcomes and satisfaction of patents of clinical nurse specialists in psychiatric mental health nursing'. *Archives of Psychiatric Nursing*, 9: 5 (1995) 240–250.

6. Taylor, D., Mace, S., Mir, S. and Kerwin, R. 'A prescription survey of the use of atypical antipsychotics for hospital inpatients in the United Kingdom'. *International Journal of Psychiatry in Clinical Practice*, 4 (2000) 41–46.

7. Gray, R. and Gourney, K. *Should Mental Health Nurses Prescribe?* Maudsley Discussion Paper Series, No. 11 (London: Institute of Psychiatry, 2001).

8. Cutliffe, J. and Campbell, P. 'Nurse prescribing power could lead nurses away from core concepts that underpin nursing'. *Mental Health Practice*, 5: 5 (2002) 14–17.

9. Department of Health. *Achieving Timely 'Simple' Discharge from Hospital* (London: HMSO, 2004).

10. Department of Health. *National Service Frame-work for Mental Health Services* (London: Department of Health, 1999).

11. Department of Health. *The NHS Plan* (London: Department of Health, 2000).

12. Department of Health. *Guidance on New Ways of Working for Psychiatrists in a Multi-disciplinary and Multi-agency Context.* Interim Report-August (2004) (London: Department of Health, 2004).

Chapter 10
School nursing perspectives

Jenny Rosalie

Introduction

This chapter will explore prescribing within a school nursing context. The current roles and responsibilities of the school nurse (SN) will be described to provide a reference point on which to base exploration and examination of the potential role of SN prescribers. This will be followed by a discussion of the possible benefits and potential problems of undertaking such a role.

School Nursing

The SN undertakes a diverse public health function in order to protect and improve the health of children and young people while at school. Their role involves a holistic approach to health improvement and protection, with interventions being aimed not only at physical but also at social and emotional health of children.

The school nursing service is non-statutory, therefore roles differ throughout the United Kingdom. There are, however, key public health elements common to most practitioners working within school health. These include:

▶ planning, implementing and evaluating health protection and promotion programmes, for example immunisation, screening programmes and health promotion campaigns
▶ assessing health needs, implementing interventions to reduce inequalities and maximise health
▶ working with school-age children and young people with medical needs such as eczema, asthma
▶ working alongside school-age children and young people with emotional or mental health difficulties

- providing young peoples services such as 'drop-in' clinics and sexual health advice
- participating in child protection partnerships with social services and other agencies
- working alongside the most vulnerable children, young people and their families
- undertaking nurse-led clinics for a range of conditions, for example enuresis, encoporesis, attention deficit hyperactivity disorder and eczema
- working alongside children and young people with special needs.

Prescribing and School Nurses

School nursing has embraced change, developing as a dynamically progressive service, which has constantly evolved to keep apace of governmental health priorities along with the health needs of communities and individuals.[1,2] This evolution has involved the SN adopting roles previously undertaken by doctors.

School nurses were initially excluded when training was commenced in 1994 for district nurses (DNs) and health visitors (HVs) to prescribe from a limited formulary, despite undertaking a role similar to that of HVs. They are now among the community specialist practitioners who may train to prescribe from the NPF, if there is a service need for them to do so. School nurses can also train to become independent and supplementary nurse prescribers if there is a clinical need.

In order for SNs to complete episodes of care, including appropriate medication supply and administration, these extended roles have been delivered using PGDs. See Chapter 18 for information relating to PGDs.

Advantages of Prescribing

There are several professional driving forces which may influence whether SNs become prescribers:

- Pressure from within – Rosalie[3] conducted a survey which reported 100 per cent of SNs surveyed were in favour of becoming prescribers.
- An evaluation carried out on behalf of the Department of Health (DH) relating to independent prescribing[4] reported nurse

prescribers' opinions that their ability to prescribe had a positive impact on the quality of patient care, enabled better use of their skills and enhanced patient access to medicines.

▶ Professional bodies – Royal College of Nursing (RCN) support SN prescribing. The RCN issued a call for every secondary school to have an SN with the power to prescribe.[5]

▶ Patient opinion may influence the need to include SNs as prescribers giving them more choice, which is at the heart of the Modernisation Agenda.

▶ The DH report '24:7 "Access to Primary Care"'[6] stressed improving access as a high priority, and considers it a key measure by which patients will judge the success of the reforming NHS. Extending nurse prescribing to SNs is in keeping with the ethos of promoting increased accessibility to treatments.

▶ When the SN is the first point of contact for the child or young person it would be an inappropriate use of resources to refer them on to their GP if the patients' needs are within the SNs' sphere of professional competence.

The research conducted for the DH[4] found patients were confident, positive and generally in favour of nurse prescribing. They reported ease of access. Obtaining prescribed medicine from a nurse rather than a doctor was considered to be a major advantage of nurse prescribing. This pattern of patient satisfaction is likely to continue with SN as prescribers. The Health Minister John Hutton stated the government's commitment to nurse prescribing in 2004:

> Extending nurse prescribing is an important part of our commitment to modernise the NHS. By breaking down traditional prescribing roles, patients can more easily access the treatment they need and are able to more fully benefit from the NHS' highly skilled workforce.[7]

Benefits to Children and Young People

School Nurses highlighted several areas of benefit for young people from independent prescribing:[3]

▶ 85 per cent of SNs considered that SN-led enuresis services would be improved.

▶ 75 per cent considered the management of community or individual infestation of *Pediculus capitis* (head lice) would improve, with SNs highlighting the potential beneficial impact on the most vulnerable children.

▶ 85 per cent felt contraceptive services would improve if the SN were able to prescribe.

▶ Bowel management and eczema management were also identified as areas that had the potential to improve.

Prescribing in Practice

Whilst prescribing from the NPF is a start for SN, there is likely to be greater benefit to school children from some SN being independent and supplementary prescribers. Supplementary prescribing facilitates service improvement in some areas for example for children with long-term conditions such as asthma and eczema. Whilst legally independent prescribers could prescribe for these conditions most SN would want to work in a prescribing partnership with GPs through the formulation of CMPs. CMPs provide parameters for safe prescribing, and, as most SN are not attached to GP surgeries, they provide an ideal mechanism for prescribing in schools, giving children and young people better access to medicines, whilst providing SN and GPs with the reassurance that they are working in partnership. Mechanisms for sharing of co-terminus records would need to be put in place. SNs trained as independent prescribers may enhance the care of children and young people with exacerbations of long-term conditions that require early treatment and in treating acute conditions that fall within their professional competence. Supplementary prescribing may be the preferred option for SNs working in the independent sector.

Community specialist prescribers are able to treat children where a diagnosis is within the remit of their role such as those with *Pediculus capitis*. Conditions that would lend themselves to independent and supplementary prescribing include those mentioned previously.

Exercise

The NPF from which V100 prescribers can prescribe autonomously is limited in its scope. Check the products included in it. Then find the children's edition of the BNF on the Internet and compare its contents.

The SN must be aware of the particular prescribing issues related to treating children under the age of 16. The BNF[8] has specific guidance on this and there is now a children's edition of the BNF.[9] SNs trained as prescribers should have access to both of these publications.

Potential Disadvantages to Prescribing

Seventy-five per cent of SNs surveyed by Rosalie[3] could identify no negative impact on care from SNs becoming prescribers. Where any potential negative impact on quality of care was envisaged, it related to issues which focussed on work load or inability to access client information.

One concern that was raised related to professional competence, due to the potential of irregular prescribing activity. The Policy Research Programme of the Department of Health[4] found that most nurses were prescribing relatively frequently, with 42 per cent prescribing between 11 and 30 items per week and 22 per cent over 30 items per week.

All nurses who currently prescribe may only do so within their level of competence.[10] The onus is on employing organisations and individual nurses to ensure their competency levels are maintained. These principles apply to all nurse prescribers including SNs. (See Chapter 19.)

A further issue which has the potential to raise concern amongst the general public is prescribing to under-sixteens, both in terms of contraception and general treatments which young people may wish to access from an SN. It is considered good practice for doctors and other health professionals to follow the criteria outlined by Lord Fraser in 1985, in the House of Lords' ruling in the case of Victoria Gillick *v.* West Norfolk and Wisbech Health Authority (1985). These are commonly known as the 'Fraser Guidelines', sometimes referred to as 'Gillick competence'.[11] Currently when supplying or administering contraception via a PGD, school nurses adhere to the Fraser Guidelines, which allow young people under the age of 16 to consent to medical treatment if they fulfil certain criteria.

The guidelines state:

- The young person understands the advice being given.
- The young person cannot be persuaded to inform their parents.

▶ The young person is likely to begin, or to continue having, sexual intercourse, with or without contraceptive treatment.

▶ Unless the young person receives contraceptive treatment, their physical or mental health, or both, are likely to suffer.

▶ The young person's best interests require them to receive contraceptive advice or treatment with or without parental consent.

Although these criteria specifically refer to contraception, the principles are deemed to apply to other treatments. Young people under the age of 16 have the same right to confidentiality as any other patient. This is enshrined in the professional code.[10]

Provision is made in Scotland by The Age of Legal Capacity (Scotland) Act 1991[12] making it lawful for doctors to provide contraceptive advice and treatment without parental consent providing certain criteria are met. Furthermore, The Sexual Offences Act 2003, ss.14 (2)–(3), 73[13] (which came into force on 1 May 2004) gives statutory protection to health professionals who provide advice about sexual matters and contraception to minors under the age of 16.

Despite young people's rights being clearly defined, some parents may remain opposed to their children receiving medication without their consent. Whilst this should not influence young people's access to services and appropriate treatment, it falls to the SN to work collaboratively wherever possible, with communities. Practitioners engage in public education to highlight young peoples' rights and assist parents to interact positively with their children in order for them to develop the attitudes and skills required in adult life.

Education and Training

At present qualified SNs training to be specialist practitioners undergo the same level of training as HVs, with increasing numbers training at masters level. In keeping with other nursing professionals, they have similar education and training needs.

In relation to independent and supplementary prescribing, the DH reported that the majority of nurses considered that the educational preparation for nurse prescribing had fully or partly met their needs.[4] They were positive and satisfied with regard to the support they had received from supervising medical practitioners.

The majority of nurses, once qualified, considered that they had been able to maintain a wide range of National Prescribing Centre competencies and two-thirds reported that they were currently receiving support or supervision for their prescribing role. However, only half of the sample reported that they had undertaken some formal CPD since qualifying. Just over 50 per cent reported that they had CPD needs in relation to nurse prescribing. The report highlighted a number of education and practice issues that have warranted further attention as the expansion of non-medical prescribing continues. There is no reason to suppose that training and education tailored to the SNs' specific needs should not reach the required standard.

Exercise

Emma Jones and her sister Emily have been sent from class with an itchy rash. You are contacted by Emma's teacher Miss Edwards from the local primary school as she suspects that Emma has chicken pox. She asks if you can visit and check this out. She is slightly apprehensive about this as she does not know the family very well and thinks Emma's aunt might be pregnant.

What are the general issues associated with this scenario? What are the prescribing issues?

Conclusion

In conclusion there was overwhelming support amongst SNs to become community nurse specialist prescribers and this is now in place. Several areas of client care have been highlighted as potentially benefiting from independent and supplementary prescribing. In particular, vulnerable children and adolescents, who may experience difficulty engaging with other professionals, may be better able to access services offered by the SN prescriber. These benefits need to be tempered against concerns with regard to education, training, CPD and resource management.

School nurses are providing the lead in many areas of public health and primary care, taking a proactive role that is responsive to need and based on best evidence. SN prescribers, along with employing organisations, will ensure that their client group receive a service which is safe, timely, appropriate and delivered by a fully trained and competent work force.

References

1. Debell, D. and Jackson, P. *School Nursing within the Public Health Agenda: A Strategy for Practice* (London: DH, 2000).

2. Department of Health. *The Health Visitor and School Nurse Development Programme: School Nurse Practice Development Resource Pack* (London: The Stationary Office, 2001).

3. Rosalie, J. School Nurses Opinion of Becoming Nurse Prescribers – A Survey. Unpublished (2005).

4. Department of Health. *An Evaluation of Extended Formulary Independent Nurse Prescribing: Executive Summary* (London: The Stationary Office, 2005).

5. RCN press briefing. *School Nurses 'Should Prescribe Contraception'.* (1999) http://news.bbc.co.uk/1/hi/health/293431.stm, accessed 3 July 2005.

6. Department of Health. *24:7 Access to Primary Care: Your Role in Sustaining Faster Access and Delivering Integrated, Unscheduled Care* (London: The Stationary Office, 2004).

7. Department of Health. *Nurses' Prescribing Powers to be Expanded Even Further* (Press Release) (London: Department of Health, 2004). http://www.dh.gov.uk/PublicationsAndStatistics/PressReleases/PressReleases Notices/fs/en?CONTENT_ID=4079503&chk=YqxsaG, accessed 9 July 2005.

8. British Medical Association/Royal Pharmaceutical Society of Great Britain. *British National Formulary.* No. 49 (London: BMA/RPSGB, March 2005).

9. British Medical Association, Royal Pharmaceutical Society of Great Britain, Royal College of Paediatrics and Child Health, Neonatal and Paediatric Pharmacists Group. *BNF for Children* (London: BMA/RPSGB/RCPCH, 2005).

10. Nursing and Midwifery Council. *Code of Professional Conduct* (London: NMC, 2002).

11. Gillick *v*. West Norfolk and Wisbech AHA [1986] AC112, [1985] 3 WLR830, [1985] 3 All ER 402, HL.

12. The Age of Legal Capacity (Scotland) Act (London: The Cabinet Office, 1991).

13. The Sexual Offences Act (London: The Cabinet Office, 2003).

Chapter 11

Community matron perspectives

Dawn Brookes

Introduction

There are many new roles for nurses emerging out of the current health care climate and government policies. Advanced nursing roles are not unfamiliar in other parts of the world,[1,2] although prescriptive authority for nurses (in advanced practice) is a relatively recent thing in the United States with only a few states adding it to their legislature.[3] It is generally agreed that advanced nursing roles involve highly autonomous practice.[4] Along with a plethora of new titles and roles comes that of the community matron[5,6] (also known as advanced primary nurse, advanced nurse practitioner). This chapter will discuss some of the issues around this new and emerging advanced nursing role. The chapter will consider in detail how independent and supplementary prescribing form a part of the toolkit required in order for this role to work in practice. Whilst focussing on one role, currently in England, there will be overlap with the roles of other nurses working in advanced practice throughout the United Kingdom and the chapter will therefore be of relevance to them.

Background

Approximately 60 per cent of adults report having some kind of long-term condition (LTC), accounting for around 17.5 million in England with over half of these having more than one condition.[5] According to the World Health Organisation (WHO), long-term conditions are set to be the leading cause of disability by 2020.[7]

The community matron forms part of the government agenda to help improve the health management of patients with LTCs through individual case management for those with highly complex or multiple LTCs.[5,6] Five per cent of patients admitted to hospital (mostly with LTCs) account for 42 per cent of acute hospital bed days.[5]

In the past, patients with LTCs have suffered from health care provision being reactive rather than proactive and it is because of this that they may end up with frequent unplanned hospital admissions. Attending numerous appointments with different health professionals can be confusing for both patients and their carers, and the patients may not feel that anyone is helping them to be in control of their conditions.[8] The government has therefore proposed a new NHS and Social Care Long-Term Conditions Model.[5] The model consists of three stages and each is vital in order for the plans to work. See Figure 11.1.

At stage 1, the infrastructure needs to be in place in order to support health care professionals in their ability to provide the best intervention at each level of care. Stage 2 gives an indication of the

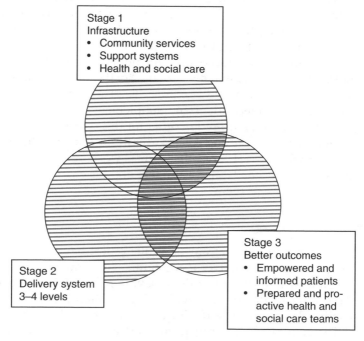

Figure 11.1 A new NHS and social care model
Source: DH

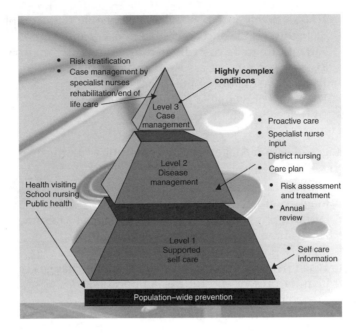

Figure 11.2 Adapted from NHS and Social Care Model Delivery System Kaiser Permanente Triangle (DH 2005)

levels of input that may be required by health professionals (see Figure 11.2) and stage 3 shows better outcomes for patients.[5]

Exercise

Identify the patient/client groups you are working with. What are the long-term conditions that these patients present with? How would prescribing assist you with their treatment? How would it assist the patients/clients? Identify any training needs (other than the prescribing course) you would require in order to be able to prescribe for these groups.

Nurses may be involved with patients at all levels of the model but community matrons will be proactively seeking out and case managing people at the top of the triangle who are estimated at being 0.5 per cent of the population. Principles of case management by community matrons are listed below:[6]

▶ To proactively focus on vulnerable people with complex LTCs.
▶ Be highly visible and accessible to users and carers.
▶ Patient care to be co-ordinated by community matron.
▶ Risks to patients are assessed and care planned.
▶ To improve quality of life of patients.
▶ To reduce preventable hospital admissions.
▶ To reduce length of hospital stay.

Stages of case management by community matrons:

▶ Manage caseloads of 50–80 people.
▶ Identify 'at risk' individuals.
▶ Perform physical, social and psychological assessment.
▶ Have authority to order tests/investigations.
▶ Identify potential risks.
▶ Teach patients/carers to recognise subtle changes in condition.
▶ Plan for present and future; support choice.
▶ Co-ordinate care.
▶ Communicate at a high level.

Community matrons will be required to have competencies in key areas including that of medicines management.

Providing an Optimum Service

The author has been involved in the development and provision of a new case management service in a PCT in England. This service has been named 'Optimum' on the basis that care given to patients with complex LTCs should be just as the name implies. In developing the service it has become apparent just how important medicines management, including independent and supplementary prescribing has been to the role of the community matron. Prescribing is an integral part of the role, as is carrying out medication reviews, including working in partnership with patients, GPs and consultants in stopping and/or altering medicines. Often, the community matron will come across the need to prescribe independently or to develop individual CMPs for supplementary prescribing[9] if this is more appropriate. A practice that has proven to be invaluable is to design disease-specific CMP templates using national and local guidelines along with current evidence-based practice and gaining approval from a local steering group which consists of senior nurses, a GP, hospital consultant and lead pharmacist. The plan is then individualised when required for a specific patient with their agreement. See examples in Appendix 2. These templates, which are based on best practice guidelines, have contributed (along with other training) towards community matrons developing the skills, pharmacological knowledge and competency required for prescribing independently for exacerbations of conditions which they come across frequently. Community matrons may be referred to as 'specialist generalists' due to the large numbers of conditions that patients present with to them. In relation to prescribing the community matron is likely to develop competency across a wide spectrum of diseases but is able to refer or seek specialist input where necessary.

Figure 11.3 shows the conditions, twelve months into the service, that people undergoing case management in the author's area present with on initial assessment. Due to the existence of nurse specialists in heart failure (HF), chronic obstructive pulmonary

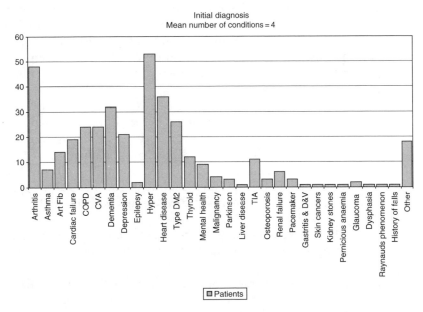

Figure 11.3 Long-term conditions people may present with on initial assessment

disease (COPD) and neurology who undertake some case management, the numbers of patients with these conditions may be fewer than in some other parts of the country.

As can be seen from Figure 11.3, many of the patients who will be on a community matron's caseload will have conditions that currently require prescribing practice which might be beyond that of the scope for independent prescribing but that fall into the remit of supplementary prescribing. Where LTCs exist in vulnerable groups such as those on the caseload of a community matron, supplementary prescribing is likely to be the preferred option for optimising treatments. The reason for this is that CMPs are evidence based and working in partnership with medical practitioners is likely to promote best practice with professionals working within agreed boundaries. Nevertheless, independent prescribing is an invaluable tool for the community matron, as particularly in relation to prompt treatment of acute exacerbations of conditions and acute illnesses that fall within their competence.

Co-morbidities

One of the major challenges facing community matrons in relation to prescribing is that of co-morbidities. The mean number of conditions found in the author's area of practice is four. There are some key areas that the community matron and any other prescriber needs to be aware of when prescribing for patients with co-morbidities, these include:

▶ Co-morbidities are more common in the elderly and many medicines need to be started at lower doses in this age group.
▶ They need to be aware of possible drug interactions.
▶ Awareness of contraindications for example amitryptilline is recommended as first-line treatment for painful peripheral neuropathy but is contraindicated in patients with recent myocardial infarction.
▶ Multiple medicines increase the risk of side effects and are often related to falls and hospitalisations in the elderly.

Figure 11.4 demonstrates how medicines management forms a large part of the community matron role. It shows that out of 1134 contacts carried out by a community matron, 438 (39 per cent)

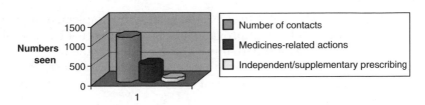

Figure 11.4 Medicines-related actions undertaken by community matrons over a period of 12 months

of them involved some form of action in relation to patients' medication. Independent and supplementary prescribing allows the community matron to prescribe for specific conditions as they arise, thereby preventing patients from waiting for prescriptions which they would often require immediately. Patients with LTCs are more likely to benefit from early intervention, adding weight to the necessity for community matrons to be prescribers.

Advanced nursing roles such as that of the community matron and those involving prescribing are in line with the aims of modernising the health service as set out in the Chief Nursing Officer (CNO) 10 key roles for nurses (England).[11]

Chief Nursing Officer (England) 10 Key Roles for Nurses

▶ To order diagnostic investigations such as pathology tests and x-rays.
▶ To make and receive referrals direct.
▶ To admit and discharge patients for specified conditions and within agreed protocols.
▶ To manage caseloads, for example diabetes, rheumatology.
▶ To run clinics, for example ophthalmology, dermatology.
▶ To prescribe medicines and treatments.
▶ To carry out a wide range of resuscitation procedures including defibrillation.
▶ To perform minor surgery.
▶ To triage patients using the latest IT developments to the most appropriate health professional.
▶ To take a lead in local health services.

In a later document,[11] the CNO describes how implementing these roles will work to improve patients' experience of the health service. For the most part, this works by reducing the waiting times for patients in that the person they see at first contact can provide appropriate care and treatment or make referrals as necessary. See Figure 11.5.

Exercise

Take a look at the CNO 10 key roles for nurses. Do these apply to your practice? List the ones that are already in place in your area of work. Explore what plans are in place locally to implement those that are missing. If you work in another part of the United Kingdom. What plans are in place for strategic nursing development?

The NHS Plan[10] sets out new ways of working for health service employees with the aim of improving the patient's experience of the NHS. Independent and supplementary prescribing for nurses and pharmacists and supplementary prescribing for other health professionals has an impact on this experience for patient's accessing the health service. Instead of unnecessary delays in treatment which may at times result in unnecessary pain or suffering and avoidable hospital admissions, the patient is treated promptly and by the health professional who is dealing with them at the time.

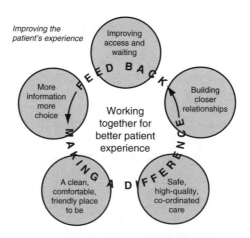

Figure 11.5 Improving the patient's experience
Source: DH

The next part of this chapter will consider some of the conditions where prescribing might be undertaken and assessment issues relating to caring for people with complex LTCs which in some instances may apply to other areas of practice. These conditions include:

- ear wax (see Chapter 5)
- infection (acute exacerbation of COPD, chest infections, urinary tract infections)
- constipation, gastro-enteritis, heartburn (see Chapter 17)
- dermatitis (see Chapter 6)
- conjunctivitis, tear deficiency (see Chapter 5)
- pain and inflammation
- palliative care (mainly non-cancer patients) (see Chapter 6).

During the winter months in particular patients on the community matron caseload are prone to infections. Many of these are viral illnesses and close observation and monitoring are required to ensure that if secondary infection occurs, treatment is prompt in order to prevent rapid deterioration and hospitalisation. One condition patients commonly present with is that of a chest infection. Where diagnosis falls within the remit of the community matron's clinical competence, treatment can be initiated early or referral to the most appropriate medical practitioner is made. Factors relating to chest infections are presented below.

Chest Infection

According to prodigy guidance, this term can be split broadly into three categories:[12]

- acute bronchitis
- exacerbation of COPD and
- community-acquired pneumonia.

Diagnosis in the community is made on clinical grounds.

Acute Bronchitis

It is often viral in origin. The patient has an acute cough with no focal chest signs. There may also be sputum, breathlessness and wheezing. It is usually a self-limiting illness with cough lasting for up to 10 days. This can persist for up to three weeks in some cases. Advice regarding symptom relief is usually all that is required. In the elderly population, however, the community matron would provide follow-up visits in order to ensure that the illness follows its normal progression and that the patient does not develop a secondary bacterial infection which would need treatment.[12]

Exacerbation of COPD

This condition presents with a worsening cough, increased breath-lessness, increased sputum and/or a change in sputum colour. NICE guidance recommends treatment if sputum is more purulent or pneumonia is suspected.[13] Treatment includes oral corticosteroid (usually prednisolone 30 mg once daily for 5–7 days), antibiotic (usually amoxicillin, 500 mg three times daily for 7 days), doxy-cycline (200 mg first day, then 100 mg once daily for 10 days) or trimethoprim (200 mg twice daily for 5–7 days) (depends also on local guidance).

Community-Acquired Pneumonia (CAP)

This presents with cough, purulent sputum (might be blood stained or rusty), dyspnoea, fever (temperature greater than 38 °C), pleuritic chest pain and systemically unwell. Chest sounds reveal crackles and pleural rub, there is dullness to percussion over the affected area and bronchial breathing is present. In the elderly the chest symptoms may not be as obvious but there is confusion, fatigue, anorexia and myalgia.[12] Due to difficulty in diagnosis Heckerling *et al.* devised a prediction tool to assist.[14] This is shown in Table 11.1.

Following diagnosis treatment is with antibiotics: amoxicillin (500 mg – 1 G three times daily for 7 days) or erythromycin (500 mg four times daily for 7 days), if no response after 48 hours add eryth-romycin (if not already started) or oxytetracycline (250–500 mg four times daily for 7 days) or doxycycline (200 mg immediately and then 100 mg once daily for 7 days). Amoxicillin or erythromycin (if penicillin allergic) are first line with erythromycin or a tetracycline added if no response after 48 hours. Hospital admission should also

Table 11.1   Tools to assist diagnosis of pneumonia

Factors	Number factors present	Probability of pneumonia where there is a 15 per cent prevalence (per cent)
• Absence of asthma	0	<1
• Heart rate >100	1	3
• Crackles	2	9
• Temperature >37.8	3	25
• Decreased breath sounds	4	51
	5	77

Source: Adapted from Heckerling *et al.*[14]

be considered if no response. Local prescribing guidelines should be consulted and any changes to national guidance.

Supplementary Prescribing

See Chapters 3 and 18 for definitions and discussions around supplementary prescribing. Much has been written around the time-consuming nature of the development of CMPs for supplementary prescribing but many practitioners have found that there are ways to make the process simpler.[15] One of the main barriers has been the lack of systems on current computer packages to generate computerised CMPs. Again, others have found ingenious ways of managing this process.[16] Generally, the use of templates around specific disease management and the individualisation of these in conjunction with patient and independent prescriber seem to be the way many practitioners have taken. It is more often than not the supplementary prescriber who formulates the plans and gains the agreement of independent prescriber and patient, and, therefore, the task has at times appeared too onerous for some. Whilst initially time-consuming, the development of disease management templates within the supplementary prescribers sphere of practice and competence brings rewards for themselves and patients later on. The process becomes less time-consuming when initiating an individualised CMP because most of the groundwork has already been carried out with reference to evidence bases and local guidelines. Caution should be continually applied to ensure that supplementary prescribers prescribe within their competence[9,17] that they always individualise CMP templates and resist the temptation to be more adventurous before they have developed competence in a specific area (see Chapter 19). In current practice the author has developed CMPs for a number of conditions, which can be found in Appendix 2.

How to Write a CMP

As previously mentioned, the advantages of CMPs is that they have to be supported by local and national guidelines. This means that those signing up to their use will be using the best evidence available rather than personal preference in relation to their prescribing practice.

In order to reduce the time taken to write CMPs it is worth spending some time developing disease templates referring to national and local guidelines. These templates can then be individualised at a later date. Blank CMP templates are available on the DH website at www.dh.gov.uk and can be used for guidance.[18] Examples of the blank templates can be found in Appendix 4 of this book.

Information that must be included in a CMP is as follows:[19]

- name of the patient
- the illness or conditions that may be treated by the supplementary prescriber
- the date on which the plan takes effect
- the date the plan is to be reviewed by the doctor (independent prescriber)
- the class or description of medicines or appliances that may be prescribed under the plan
- any restrictions or limitations as to the strength or dose of medicine to be prescribed
- a reference to published national or local guidelines – These must clearly identify the range of the relevant medicinal products to be used in the treatment. The CMP should draw attention to the relevant part of the guideline which should be easily accessible
- relevant allergies, known sensitivities of the patient

- arrangements for notification of suspected or known reactions to a medicine; suspected or known reactions to any other medicine the patient is taking at the same time; incidents occurring with an appliance which might lead, might have led or has led to death of serious deterioration of the health of the patient
- circumstances when the supplementary should refer back to the independent prescriber.

Decisions need to be made as to what is to be included in the CMP:

1. Names of specific medicines or broader terms such as 'ACE inhibitors' to be used.
2. Specific dose schedules or broader terms such as 'titrate according to BNF'.
3. Other areas such as secondary prevention to be included. For instance in the case of diabetes is a Statin to be included according to national guidance?
4. Is the CMP going to be signed by one independent prescriber or a number of them. Whilst having more than one may save time in re-writing a CMP if the independent prescriber is sick, on annual leave or leaves, there are issues surrounding patient safety where there are a number of independent prescribers and who takes overall responsibility?
5. Is the CMP to be signed by one supplementary prescriber or more than one. An example might include specialist nurses in a heart failure clinic. If one is on holiday, the patient can still be seen by others in the team but they will not be able to alter medication if they are not signed up the the CMP.
6. Where co-terminus records are not available, patients' current medication should be included. In practice this becomes unwieldy and impractical as when new medication is added, in theory the CMP should be re-written. It is good practice to obtain an up-to-date medication list from the surgery prior to visiting a patient at home and as long as this is always done, the current medication might be excluded from the CMP.

Once these factors have been decided it is still vitally important to make patient-specific alterations to a plan before initiating it in practice.

Conclusion

Medicines management, including prescribing, is an invaluable part of the community matron's toolkit. This will apply to many other nurses working in specialist or advanced roles. Whilst still being an onerous task to keep up to date with changing regulations and legislation, the value to patients and the rewards for health care professionals of individual job satisfaction cannot be underestimated. Prescribing is an appropriate use of the knowledge and skills of many health care professionals and can only be of benefit to the NHS overall. Community matrons case manage relatively small numbers of patients with highly complex LTCs and are, therefore, best placed to carry out medication reviews and to prescribe for these patients in many instances. Supplementary prescribing partnerships for community matrons may include hospital consultants as well as GPs. Many patients have anecdotally expressed satisfaction at being treated promptly and by the health care professional that they see the most. GPs can be satisfied that they may have fewer interruptions to surgery in order to prescribe or sign a prescription on behalf of another health care professional.

References

1. Jones, M. Role development and effective practice in specialist and advanced practice roles in acute hospital settings: Systematic review and meta-synthesis. *Journal of Advanced Nursing*, 49:2 (2005) 191–209.

2. Daly, W. and Carnwell, R. Nursing roles and levels of practice: A framework for differentiating between elementary, specialist and advancing nursing practice. *Journal of Clinical Nursing*, 12:2 (2003) 158–167.

3. Phillips, S. A comprehensive look at the legislative issues affecting advanced nursing practice. *Nurse Practitioner*, 30:1 (2005) 14–47.

4. Bryant-Lukosius, D., DiCenso, A., Browne, G. and Pinelli, J. Advanced practice nursing roles: Development, implementation and evaluation. *Journal of Advanced Nursing*, 48:5 (2004) 519–529.

5. DH. *Supporting People with Long term Conditions: An NHS and Social Care Model to Support Local Innovation and Integration* (London: DH, January 2005).

6. DH. *Supporting People with Long term Conditions: Liberating the Talents of Nurses Who Care for People with Long Term Conditions* (London: DH, February 2005).

7. WHO. *World Health Report 2002: Reducing Risks, Promoting Healthy Life.* www.who.int/whr/2002, accessed 31/05/05.

8. Billingham, K. Front Line Framework. *Nursing Standard*, 19:25 (2005) 16–17.

9. DH. *Supplementary Prescribing by Nurses, Pharmacists, Chiropodists/ Podiatrists, Physiotherapists and Radiographers within the NHS in England: A Guide for Implementation* (London: DH, May 2005).

10. DH. *The NHS Plan* (London: DH, 2000).

11. Chief Nursing Officer. *Developing Key Roles for Nurses and Midwives: A Guide for Managers* (2002). www.dh.gov.uk/Publicationsandstatistics/ Publications/PublicationsPolicyandGuidan ce/, accessed 31/05/05.

12. Prodigy. *Prodigy Guidance: Chest Infections.* 2nd edition (London: The Stationary Office, 2005).

13. NICE. Chronic obstructive pulmonary disease. Clinical guideline12 (NICE, 2004). www.nice.org.uk, accessed 27/10/05.

14. Heckerling, P.S., Tape, T.G., Wigton, R.S., Hissong, K.K., Leikin, J.B., Ornato, J.P., Cameron, J.L. and Racht, E.M. Clinical prediction rule for pulmonary infiltrates. *Annals of Internal Medicine*, 113 (1990) 664–670.

15. Langridge, P. Extended independent and supplementary prescribing: An update. *Paediatric Nursing*, 16:3 (2004) 21 23.

16. Belton, J. Developing a computer based clinical management plan for supplementary prescribing. *Nurse Prescribing*, 3:2 (2005) 76–78.

17. Brookes, D. Selecting and developing extended and supplementary nurse prescriber. *Nurse Prescribing*, 2:5 (2004) 212–216.

18. DH. Clinical Management Plan Templates. www.dh.gov.uk, accessed 28/10/05.

19. DH. Clinical Management Plans (CMPs). www.dh.gov.uk/PolicyAndGuidance/ MedicinesPharmacyAndIndustry/, accessed 15/07/05.

Part III

Allied health professionals and supplementary prescribing

Chapter 12
Pharmacy and prescribing

Angela Alexander

Introduction

The announcement made in November 2002 that pharmacists were to become supplementary prescribers was welcomed by the profession. Prescribing is a natural extension of the pharmacist's role. They undertake four years of undergraduate study and one year of postgraduate training before registration. Pharmacists spend more time studying drugs, their actions and uses than any other health care professional. One of the 10 key roles for a pharmacist is 'to prescribe medicines and to monitor clinical outcomes'.[1] And yet despite this, the number of pharmacists who have qualified to become supplementary prescribers has been below the target set by the Department of Health (see Chapter 4). It was proposed that 1000 pharmacists would be trained as supplementary prescribers by the of end 2004; in fact there were about 400 pharmacists qualified to prescribe at that time out of a total of 36,000 practising pharmacists on the register in Great Britain.

This situation may change with the announcement by the Secretary of State that, from spring 2006, pharmacists will be able to train as independent prescribers, and be able to prescribe any licensed medicine for any medical condition, with the exception of CDs.[2] Pharmacists feel they have always been independently prescribing albeit not for the NHS. The supply of medicines classified as Pharmacy (P) medicines from registered premises under the supervision of a pharmacist which is often referred to as an 'over the counter' sale is perhaps more appropriately called 'counter prescribing'. The process requires assessment of the patient's symptoms, an element of differential diagnosis, and then choice of a medication appropriate for the patient and their condition.

The major pharmaceutical organisations all supported independent prescribing from the whole of the BNF with no restrictions on the conditions for which a pharmacist could prescribe.[3] The emphasis of the responses was that pharmacists would be expected to prescribe within their area of competence or scope of practice; pharmacists should recognise that they have prescribing responsibilities rather than prescribing rights.

Developing the Role and Building a Business Case

To some extent pharmacy shares the same constraints in developing the role as does nursing, but in other aspects it faces different challenges related to the historical location of the pharmacist and the perceived extent of patient contact. Nurses are in the right location and have good patient contact but they have less knowledge of drugs. Pharmacists have the knowledge, but have been perceived as having less patient contact. It is therefore necessary to develop a business case for pharmacist prescribing.

The key elements of building a business case can be based on the aims of supplementary prescribing in the implementation guidance published by the Department of Health in February 2003.[4] It said supplementary prescribing was intended to provide patients with quicker and more efficient access to medicines, and to make the best use of the skills of pharmacists. It stated that, over time, supplementary prescribing was also likely to reduce doctors' workloads, freeing up their time to concentrate on patients with more complicated conditions and who need more complex treatments. In building a case for pharmacist prescribing it therefore helps to identify the clinical need and benefit to patients, the views from patients, medical and nursing staff and have a statement of support from the independent prescriber. It is necessary to find out what the organisation's targets are and how pharmacist prescribing might help to achieve them. Particular risk areas, highlighted through either local or national incidents, may support the case for pharmacist input.

In secondary care, pharmacists are already involved in many activities which are effectively prescribing. Pharmacists arrange for the supply of take-home medicines for patients being discharged, usually by transcription of an original direction made by a doctor. Pharmacists have also been running anticoagulant clinics and adjusting doses. Building a business case for prescribing in such cases is therefore easier. Initially it may only be possible to obtain limited funding, but with agreed review and report mechanisms the impact can be monitored and a case made for extension.

Case study 1

This case study provides a good example of a business case for the development of pharmacist prescribing. A high-risk medicines monitoring service was set up by the Bart's and the London NHS Trust in response to the death of a patient taking oral methotrexate daily rather than weekly.

The High-Risk Medicines Monitoring Service targets drugs that pose a risk in this area such as methotrexate, azathioprine, mercaptopurine and sulphasalazine used in, for example, gastroenterology and rheumatology. The focus is on monitoring, patient education, GP support and communication across the interface. The role of the pharmacist is to manage these high-risk medicines by providing patient education, advice and support, monitoring for potential side effects, advising on dose alterations, and supporting GPs in the repeat-prescribing process by improved communication across the interface.

For example, in the inflammatory bowel disease (IBD) clinic, clinically stable follow-up patients are not routinely seen by a gastroenterologist. The pharmacist undertakes:

- questioning for IBD symptoms
- taking a medication history
- questioning for medicines-related side-effects
- discussion of therapy
- provision of information sheets and monitoring booklet
- counselling on side-effects and drug interactions, lifestyle, dose alterations and prophylactic medication
- taking blood samples.

The benefits have been

- improved patient experience
- increased clinic capacity by up to 20 per cent
- minimising of risk
- patient education
- improved communication
- recommendations on medication.

Contact: Sasha Beresford, Department of Pharmacy, Bart's and the London NHS Trust
Email: Sasha.Beresford@bartsandthelondon.nhs.uk

For community pharmacists, the key to funding is to identify where prescribing will benefit GPs and meet patient need. It is important for the proposal to fit in with the Primary Care Organisation

(PCO) priorities, locality strategic plans and health needs. In order to justify the support and training for a pharmacist to become a prescriber many PCOs want to receive an outline proposal, showing potential benefits, giving details of costings, time allocations, and how the service will be delivered and evaluated.

Exercise

Build a business case for pharmacist prescribing in your area of practice. Remember to consider the needs of patients, other health care professionals and the commissioners of the service.

Benefits and Risks of Pharmacist Prescribing

With any new service it is necessary to consider the strengths and weaknesses, benefits and risks. The Royal West Sussex NHS Trust and Western Sussex PCT[5] stated that the benefits must include improved patient care but other benefits will vary depending on the needs of the local health care economy and could include:

- improved access and reduced delays for patients
- clear specific treatment plans for patients
- help in addressing the problems associated with junior doctors' hours
- help in addressing a shortage in GPs
- encouraging the treatment of some conditions by community pharmacists
- reducing waste by allowing pharmacists to repeat prescribe
- improved drug-related information on discharge for GPs and community pharmacists
- greater job satisfaction for professionals undertaking this advanced practice
- improved training of junior doctors in prescribing.

They also identified the following risks, which will impact on the development and continuation of the role of pharmacist as prescriber:

- shortages of appropriate pharmacists to undertake these roles
- inability to release staff to train
- shortage of mentors

- training of staff without a role to use their newfound skills
- individuals losing their own professional uniqueness
- lack of funding to provide such services (particularly in primary care).

It is important that these risks are addressed for a service to be sustainable.

Exercise

Are the risks listed above relevant to your area of practice? How do you intend to minimise them as part of a risk management strategy?

Preparation for Pharmacist Prescribing

In addition to the business case a considerable amount of background work is needed in preparation for pharmacist prescribing. It is important to have the support of the key managers and stakeholders. Other health care professionals and the appropriate directorate leads need to be educated on the process of pharmacist prescribing. It is also necessary to prepare the workplace for the training required for pharmacist prescribing. Both the student and their colleagues need to know the course workload and the portfolio requirements. A policy should be agreed on 'protected' study time.

One of the practical aspects of implementing pharmacist prescribing is to ensure that it is encompassed in the organisation's medicines policy. Existing documentation may need to be amended to incorporate developments in prescribing. Representation by pharmacist prescribers on drugs and therapeutics committees or medicines management committees may also be appropriate.

The sustainability of pharmacist prescribing needs to be addressed as part of the long-term development. Succession planning is an important issue which needs to be addressed. At present many of the models of pharmacist prescribing are based on the individual who has trained to become a prescriber. Having a patient-centred service based on one individual is not really sustainable. It is therefore important that more pharmacists are trained to maintain the service.

Case study 2 shows how a service model for pharmacist prescribing has been designed around the patient journey for surgical patients.

Case study 2

A service model for supplementary prescribing pharmacists working with surgical patients has been developed by the West-Hertfordshire Hospitals NHS Trust. Pharmacists had been involved in surgical preoperative assessment clinics for a few years and the flow chart below outlines how the service is being adapted to operate now with a pharmacist as a supplementary prescriber.

Patient presents to GP
↓
GP makes provisional diagnosis and refers patient to surgeon
↓
Diagnosis by surgeon and decision to operate (for example gall bladder surgery)
↓
Referral made by surgeon to pharmacist in pre-surgery clinic. This is done by a note in the patient record that is supported by a pre-agreed CMP and a trust protocol
↓
Patient comes to pharmacist's pre-admission clinic 1–2 weeks prior to surgery. CMP completed. Peri-operative medication prescribed on drug chart. Patient counselled regarding appropriate medication to stop prior to admission. Discharge prescription drafted for routine post-operative medications. Drug history completed by pharmacist. All regular medication transcribed on drug chart (not signed). Patient is told to inform surgical team on admission if any change to medication occurs prior to surgery for team to amend pre-written chart. Copy of CMP and drug history kept in medical notes.
↓
Patient admitted for surgery.
Doctor checks and signs patient's regular medication and adds any new changes.
↓
Post surgery, peri-operative therapy continues to be monitored and prescribed by pharmacist according to hospital protocols and CMP. Discharge medication for pain control is prescribed as required according to CMP and patient's requirement. Regular medication not prescribed on discharge. Any changes are communicated to GP.
↓
Follow-up – Patient contacted by pharmacist during the week following discharge regarding pain control.

Contact: Rekha Shah, Pharmacy Department, West-Herts Hospitals NHS Trust
Email: Rekha.Shah@whht.nhs.uk

The transfer of prescribing responsibilities from one clinical area to another is also an issue for consideration when, for example, a registered prescriber switches clinical area to a new patient group, or a prescriber is recruited into a new position. There needs to be consideration of whether the pharmacist's competence is a matter for their own professional responsibility or whether organisations should have governance frameworks that require an additional period of supervised practice in the new area.

The Barts and the London NHS Trust have a the Non-Medical Prescribing Policy,[6] which states that supplementary prescribers joining the Trust and those planning to extend their prescribing to a new clinical specialty must undertake a further 12 days practice under the supervision of the independent prescriber with whom they will be working. The policy suggests that a reflective practice diary is completed during this time to ensure training needs are identified and met. The independent prescriber must also confirm the competence of the supplementary prescriber to carry out their role before prescribing commences.

In community pharmacy, pharmacist prescribers could potentially be responsible for both prescribing and dispensing medicines. The Department of Health has suggested that they would normally expect separation of prescribing and dispensing roles where this is feasible, in keeping with the principles of safety and clinical and corporate governance. However, they have said that in the context of supplementary prescribing, dispensing and prescribing need not necessarily be separated, provided clear accountability arrangements are in place to assure patient safety and probity.[7] They suggest that where the two roles do co-exist, a final accuracy check must be carried out by another person, ideally a qualified pharmacy technician.

Exercise

In your area of practice what preparation is needed for pharmacist prescribing? Who do you need to talk to and what processes need to be in place?

Competencies and Training

At the beginning of 2006, prescribing courses for pharmacists were available from 34 higher education institutes in the United Kingdom. It is anticipated that some of the knowledge elements of training to become a prescriber will be incorporated into the undergraduate training of pharmacy students. However, the skills to become competent to be a pharmacist prescriber will still be assessed after a suitable period of supervised practice some years after registration. See Chapter 12 for details relating to pharmacist prescribing training.

Legal Liability

The legal liability of becoming a prescriber needs to be considered prior to commencement of the service. All employees working for the NHS are covered by their respective NHS organisation. The extent of vicarious liability held by an NHS Trust for prescribers may be subject to certain criteria being met, such as working with the approval of the line manager and within the legal framework of the role, their CMP, and within Trust policies. It is therefore important that an individual's responsibilities are outlined in their job description prior to commencement of prescribing.

Some pharmacists have also taken out additional personal professional indemnity insurance. This could be of value in obtaining independent legal representation, for example, if they ever have to defend an action that they have taken that is outside normally accepted practice. For community pharmacists, who are independent practitioners, there are various companies who provide indemnity insurance for their practice as pharmacists. At the time of writing the indemnity could be extended to pharmacists who have qualified as supplementary prescribers for no additional premium. This may be reviewed as the service gets underway and the risk can be evaluated more fully.

Contractual and Governance Arrangements in Primary Care

Contractual arrangements for supplementary prescribing in primary and community care have been developed by some PCOs.

Brent tPCT has a Policy for Supplementary Prescribers whether they are employed by the tPCT or are Independent Contractors.[8] It suggests that a Service Level Agreement (SLA) is set up between the community pharmacist prescriber, the GP practice and the PCT. In addition to the standard requirements for supplementary prescribing the SLA should include annual clinical audits in specific areas such as ensuring that prescribing is in line with the CMP. It also suggests that any patient surveys should include a section that explores the patient's experience of pharmacist prescribing.

Brent requires pharmacist prescibers to be included in the Controls Assurance programme for risk management and patient safety and adhere to the PCT clinical governance procedures. Pharmacists are required to provide validation of ongoing CPD and evidence of indemnity insurance. The level of access to patients' notes and details of who will be responsible for updating notes also forms part of the SLA. Finally, the pharmacist supplementary prescriber must state how his/her dispensing and prescribing responsibilities are going to be managed to avoid any conflict of interest.

The RPSGB have developed a Clinical Governance Framework for pharmacist prescribers and organisations commissioning or participating in pharmacist prescribing.[9] It has been developed from two distinct viewpoints. First, from an organisational perspective it looks at the components of clinical governance and what might need to be put in place in order to support clinical governance of pharmacist prescribing. Such organisations include PCOs, NHS Trusts, the private and voluntary health care sector and all organisations that employ pharmacist prescribers providing care to both NHS and non-NHS patients. Secondly, from an individual pharmacist prescribers' point of view, the guideline provides some suggested indicators of good practice for pharmacist prescribing and examples of good clinical governance practice relating to prescribing.

Exercise

If you are a pharmacist prescriber, what clinical governance procedures do you have in place to support your prescribing role? If you are an employer or commissioner of the services of a pharmacist prescriber what procedures would you expect to be in place?

What evidence will be provided that standards are being met?

Potential for Pharmacist Prescribing

The areas where there is potential for pharmacist prescribing vary according to location. For PCO or practice-based pharmacists it has been suggested that they are employed on a sessional basis by GP practices to manage long-term conditions where a pharmacist's expertise would be valuable. They could undertake medication review clinics, participate in diabetes and hypertension clinics and make domiciliary visits for medication reviews. Case study 3 exemplifies this in action.

Case study 3

A practice pharmacist in the Rowley Regis and Tipton PCT working with six GP practices has developed a service as a supplementary prescriber for the treatment of hypertension. A small number of nurse supplementary prescribers were already trained in PCT but their skills were, in the main, underused. Initially two practices opted to include the development of pharmacist-led hypertension clinics in their objectives under criteria MM6 of the Quality and Outcome Framework (QOF).

The clinic was initially scheduled for one session every other week, with ten appointments of twenty minutes per session. Close liaison with the practice managers was necessary to resolve practical difficulties. GPs are encouraged to refer newly or recently diagnosed patients into clinic. Patients with a recorded diagnosis of hypertension who have not been seen within 12 months are contacted and recalled. Patients attend for an introductory appointment where the concept of supplementary prescribing is explained using an explanatory leaflet. Consent is obtained to prepare a CMP, which is then agreed with a GP of the patient's choice prior to the next appointment. Medicines are then prescribed by the pharmacist as appropriate.

Factors which have been found to ease the transition of patients into the clinic include an explanation of the clinic and the supplementary prescribers' role by the referring GP, provision of adequate supplies of existing treatment to cover the first clinic appointment and involvement of the patient in the process. Several of the clinics are now running weekly to satisfy growing demand.

GPs have been receptive to the clinic but there have been variable rates and suitability of referrals. Supplementary prescribing has not always been the most suitable option for the patient.

Contact: Richard Thompson, Rowley Regis and Tipton PCT
Email: richard.thompson3@nhs.net

When community pharmacists achieve networked access to patient records, as proposed in the NHS Programme for IT there will be more opportunities for prescribing, for example generating repeat prescriptions for some LTCs. In line with PCO-identified priorities, pharmacists could also manage and prescribe for cohorts of patients in the community with LTCs such as cardiovascular disease, asthma or osteoporosis.

Particular areas where hospital pharmacist prescribing is perceived as valuable include:

- clozapine clinics
- anticoagulant clinics
- intensive care units
- total parenteral nutrition (TPN) prescribing
- treatment requiring therapeutic drug monitoring
- day surgery for pain control and antibiotic cover.

Hospital pharmacists working with consultant teams can also assist in adjusting medication and prescribing on patient's discharge. Pharmacist prescribers also have a role in training junior doctors to improve their prescribing. Case study 4 demonstrates a multi-disciplinary team approach involving both nurse and pharmacist prescribers in secondary care.

Case study 4

Potential areas for the development of pharmacist prescribing within the cardiac care group at King's College Hospital were initially identified as:

- anticoagulation
- anti-anginal therapy
- comprehensive risk reduction clinics – aspirin, ACEI, beta-blocker, statin
- heart failure – especially for dose-titration programmes
- lipid management programmes
- compliance clinics/medication review.

The development of a new specialist heart failure service presented the first opportunity for pharmacist prescribing within the Trust. In the traditional management of heart failure (prior to establishment of the clinic) patients

Case study 4 cont'd

were seen at intervals of up to 6 months by the cardiology team. Between these visits the patients were managed primarily by the GP. Lack of intensive follow-up frequently resulted in a failure to achieve therapeutic targets and a lack of structured support for patients. The consequence was poor compliance, failure of symptom control, recurrent re-admissions to hospital and high mortality.

In the new multi-disciplinary team approach at King's College Hospital, diagnosis is confirmed on the first visit by consultant cardiologist and then further management, including prescribing, is delegated to a nurse consultant and specialist pharmacist. There is intensive clinic supervision until symptoms are controlled and drug therapy optimised, followed by 3 to 6 monthly reviews as necessary. Patients are therefore diagnosed by an independent prescriber, with responsibility for follow-up delegated to both the nurse and pharmacist supplementary prescribers.

While both nurse and pharmacist are supplementary prescribers, their primary roles within the clinic are as following:
For nurse consultant:

- initial assessment
- tests and investigations
- physical examination
- educating patients on HF pathology
- lifestyle advice
- social issues/psychology
- dealing with carers
- co-ordinating clinic visits
- tele-clinics.

For pharmacist:

- drug histories
- medication review
- optimising dosing
- tailoring drug therapy
- monitoring response to drug therapy
- dealing with adverse effects
- providing patient information and GP letters.

Contact: Helen Williams, Pharmacy Department, King's College Hospital
Email: helen.williams@kingsch.nhs.uk

Exercise

Case study 4 shows how pharmacist and nurse prescribers can work together in a team. How would this work in your area of practice?

Supplementary Prescribing and Clinical Management Plans

The introduction of independent prescribing by pharmacists has raised discussion about the future of supplementary prescribing based on clinical management plans (CMPs). It is agreed there is still a place for it, particularly in the care of patients who may have more than one prescriber or where treatment is complex and a defined treatment plan would be of benefit.

Writing of CMPs is seen as a key role for the pharmacist prescriber. Whilst CMPs need to be simple documents, they also have to be broad enough to allow supplementary prescribers to practice efficiently. For example, for heart failure, the CMP might include not only symptom control and the optimising of outcomes but also hypertension management, secondary prevention of ischaemic heart disease, anti-anginal therapy, management of atrial fibrillation, obesity and even sexual dysfunction. See Appendix 2 for examples of CMPs.

For patients with co-morbidities it may be difficult to present all the options for supplementary prescribing within one CMP. Some pharmacist prescribers have found it necessary to use generic bite-sized CMP templates for individual problems then build them into individual CMPs which are agreed and kept in the patient's records, often electronically in paperless practices. The National Electronic Library for Medicines website has a section 'Extending Prescribing' which contains a wide range of resources to support the implementation of supplementary prescribing and has been used for the sharing of CMPs.[10] An online resource for CMPs has also been set up.[11]

Conclusion

The introduction of independent prescribing by pharmacists opens up a new approach to care. It gives patients quicker access to the medicines they need and maximises benefit to NHS services, by making better and more flexible use of the

Conclusion cont'd

skills of pharmacists. It also opens up the possibility of private prescribing outside of the NHS. The extent to which all aspects of pharmacists prescribing will be provided by pharmacists, commissioned by the NHS and accepted by the public is speculative at this stage. It could, however, contribute to a radical change to the current provision of health care.

References

1. Department of Health. *A Vision for Pharmacy in the New NHS* (London: Department of Health, 2003).

2. Department of Health. *Nurse and Pharmacist Prescribing Powers Extended*. Press release, 10 November 2005.

3. News feature. 'Is a full formulary the best option for pharmacists prescribing independently?' *Pharmacy Journal*, 274 (2005) 607.

4. Department of Health. *Supplementary Prescribing by Nurses and Pharmacists with the NHS in England: A Guide for Implementation* (London: Department of Health, 2003).

5. Royal West Sussex NHS Trust and Western Sussex PCT. *Grasping the Opportunities for Nurse and Pharmacist Supplementary Prescribers* (Sussex: Royal West Sussex NHS Trust and Western Sussex PCT, 2003).

6. Bart's and the London NHS Trust. *Policy and Guidelines for Non-Doctor Prescribing (Including Supplementary Prescribing and Extended Nurse Prescribing* (2004). www.druginfozone.nhs.uk, accessed 18/02/06.

7. Department of Health. *Supplementary Prescribing by Nurses, Pharmacists, Chiropodists/Podiatrists, Physiotherapists and Radiographers within the NHS in England: A Guide for Implementation* (London: Department of Health, May 2005).

8. Brent tPCT. *Policy for Supplementary Prescribers whether Employed by the tPCT or as Independent Contractors*. 2004. www.druginfozone.nhs.uk accessed 18/02/06.

9. Royal Pharmaceutical Society of Great Britain. *Clinical Governance Framework for Pharmacist Prescribers and Organisations Commissioning or Participating in Pharmacist Prescribing* (London: Royal Pharmaceutical Society of Great Britain, October 2005). http://www.rpsgb.org.uk/pdfs/clincgovframework pharm.pdf, accessed 18/02/06.

10. National electronic Library for Medicines (NeLM) http://www.druginfozone.
    nhs.uk, accessed 18/02/06.

11. Clinical Management Plans Online. http://www.cmponline.info/, accessed
    18/02/06.

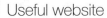 Useful website

Royal Pharmaceutical Society of
Great Britain

www.rpsgb.org.uk/members
www.rpsgb.org.uk/pdfs/
pharmprescriberpack.pdf

Chapter 13

Physiotherapy and prescribing

Penny Robinson

Historical Background

The profession of physiotherapy has its origins in the formation of the Institution of Trained Masseurs in 1894. The key modality of practice in 1894 was massage but within ten years, exercise and electrotherapy were added. The Chartered Society for Massage and Medical Gymnastics was incorporated by Royal Charter in 1920, and then in 1942 the organisation was renamed the Chartered Society of Physiotherapy (CSP). The prime purpose of the Institute and later the Chartered Society was to set up and develop educational and practice standards, which continues to this day.

Physiotherapy

The Curriculum Framework for qualifying programmes in physiotherapy published by the CSP in 2002 describes physiotherapy as:

'A health care profession concerned with function and movement and maximising patient potential. It uses physical approaches to promote, maintain and restore physical, psychological and social wellbeing, taking into account variations in health status. It is science-based, committed to extending, applying, evaluating and reviewing the evidence that underpins and informs its practice and delivery. The exercise of clinical judgement and informed interpretation is at its core.'[1]

'The profession adopts an holistic approach to the management of patients/clients, which utilises and enhances the body's natural healing mechanisms.'[1]

Physiotherapy has developed considerably over the past hundred years and continues to explore and identify new modalities and interventions which will be of benefit to patients.

Several key factors have led to the development of the profession:

▶ The choice, range and application of different treatment techniques, and modalities – themselves brought about by changing and improving technology, research and development.
▶ Practitioner innovation – leading to the development of new approaches, their rigorous testing and subsequent adoption by the profession at large.
▶ The evolution of services for new client groups and more generally the increasing expectations of clients.

Treatments

Although traditionally the profession has practised physical approaches to treatment such as manual techniques, exercise and the application of heat, cold and light, the practice of the profession has been within the orthodox care sector. It has, on occasions, been called the 'orthodox alternative' profession in that what could be seen as alternative or complementary treatments (as they are now known) are practised within the orthodox medical environment of hospitals. It is interesting to note that a number of complementary therapies have, in the last few years, been incorporated into the scope of practice of the profession.

These include:

▶ acupuncture
▶ reflex therapy
▶ aromatherapy
▶ cranial osteopathy.

Medicines Use and Prescribing

The profession has also been aware of and used medicines to facilitate and improve the outcome of physiotherapeutic interventions. This use of medicines has occurred for a number of years and includes the use of bronchodilators such as salbutamol when treating patients with respiratory conditions, anaesthetics and steroids when treating joint and spinal problems and to increase mobility. The use of medicines in this manner was governed by what was called patient protocols and in more recent years by the employment of PGDs. (See Chapter 18.)

Alongside the development of the use of medicines, as an adjunct to treatment, physiotherapists have also extended their scope to include the injection of medicines where indicated.

This was developed for two key reasons:

1. The development of the 'Extended Scope practitioner' (ESP) in the late 1990s where physiotherapists, initially working in orthopaedic out-patients, were working in a variety of ways, triaging and treating patients on behalf of orthopaedic surgeons. Following on from this a paper published in January 2001[2] outlined the role undertaken by ESPs in Stockport and reported that they were undertaking injection therapy using a supply of local anaesthetic and steroids for the administration of intra- and extra-articular steroid injections. This activity had been undertaken by the use of PGDs.
2. In both the private and NHS sectors many physiotherapists treat a large number of patients with musculoskeletal problems including acute injuries. As part of the holistic approach to treatment, physiotherapists recognise that the condition will either be alleviated or treatment enhanced by the use of an intra- or extra-articular injection of anaesthetic or steroid. To facilitate this, a referral back to the GP would normally take place. Increasingly the practice has developed that a GP will prescribe the relevant medicine, advising the patient to obtain this from a local pharmacist and then return to the physiotherapist who will administer it.

These developments in practice clearly demonstrate all the factors identified by the Department of Health[3] and the profession in relation to the need to extend the role of physiotherapists. This includes medicines being prescribed to improve care and outcomes, as in this way, services available to patients are increased along with improved access times.

The profession watched with interest the developments in respect of nurse prescribing from the outcome of the Cumberlege Report[4] to the Review of the Medicines Report[5] chaired by Dr June Crown. The CSP, following discussion with the membership, responded to a consultation relating to prescribing and argued that physiotherapists should be able to administer and prescribe certain medicines.

The profession's response included the following key points:

▶ Physiotherapeutic care of a patient can be facilitated by timely prescriptions and administration of a medicine and this ability should be given to the physiotherapy profession.
▶ Prescribing would maximise effective and timely use of resources.
▶ It is vital that any change enables therapists to prescribe, supply and administer medicines in a safe and competent manner. This would entail recognised post-qualification education being put in place to enable therapists who so wish to embrace this extension of practice.
▶ Extension of education and training for physiotherapists to prescribe for specific conditions from a restricted formulary could be an interim measure – however, this would be a short-term approach and would not empower efficacious prescribing as new drugs become available. Therefore any restriction by either condition or medicine is not desirable.

The second Crown Report[5] was extremely helpful in that it legitimised current practice regarding the use of PGDs and Patient Specific Directions (PSDs), therefore establishing the role of physiotherapists as suppliers and administrators of appropriate medicines to enhance and support physiotherapeutic interventions.

The profession has taken advantage of this and both PGDs and PSDs are used across the United Kingdom to facilitate the use of medication for patients in a number of areas including accident and emergency departments, walk-in centres, private practices as well as acute surgical and medical wards.

The report also clarified and defined the types of prescribers, for example independent and supplementary. The CSP took the opportunity to respond to the Crown II Report to identify and promote that:

▶ Physiotherapists could be either independent or supplementary practitioners – this would depend on their education, training and individual circumstances.

▷ There should be no restriction on the medicines available for new prescribers; any restriction would relate to the education and training of the individual clinician.
▷ There must be full access to details of patients' records and medication for the physiotherapist to ensure patient safety.
▷ The involvement of the CSP to set training guidelines was essential.

With the enactment of the Health and Social Care Act 2001, the ability was given for physiotherapists to be granted supplementary prescribing rights.

Currently physiotherapists have permission to become supplementary prescribers together with podiatry and radiography colleagues.[6,7] A core curriculum has been recommended building on that for nurses and pharmacists and a set of competencies have been developed in collaboration with the National Prescribing Centre.[7] Both the core curriculum and the competency framework involved considerable input from chartered physiotherapists.

Courses will require validation by the Health Professions Council (HPC) to allow practitioners to record their qualification. See Chapter 2 for more information regarding training.

Although the profession does not expect a large number of physiotherapists to extend their practice to include supplementary prescribing, there are significant groups of patients who could benefit. These include patients with LTCs whose main clinical contact is with a physiotherapist. Following are examples of these patients:

▷ Patients with Long-term respiratory conditions such as COPD. The medicines most likely to be prescribed in these situations would include bronchodilators such as salbutamol, ipratropium bromide and steroid inhalers such as beclomethasone, other medicines might include oral steroids for those with expertise in this area.
▷ Patients with neurological conditions such as multiple sclerosis (MS) and Parkinson's disease (PD). Physiotherapists may need to titrate doses of muscle relaxants such as Baclofen in order to carry out physiotherapy. Another treatment may include Botulinum A Toxin which is widely used to reduce spasticity in patients with stroke or cerebral palsy. Analgesics could also feature with this group of patients.

- Patients with musculoskeletal conditions including osteoarthritis and rheumatoid arthritis. The wide spectrum of anti-inflammatory medicines could be prescribed by physiotherapists in these conditions including NSAIDs or steroids. Again, analgesia could feature as an adjunct to treatment.
- Patients with urinary and faecal incontinence as well as the effects of constipation. They are often treated in the long term by physiotherapists and physiotherapy. A wide range of medicines can be used in these situations.
- Patients suffering from chronic pain caused by a number of underlying conditions. They are often seen in the long term by physiotherapists. The objective of these interventions being to reduce dependency and improve mobility and function; paracetamol and its derivatives together with opioids could be prescribed (although at present physiotherapists will not be able to prescribe CDs). NSAIDs and some antiepileptic medicines can also be used in the treatment of chronic pain.

Many patients are likely to be taking medication for their condition which could require dose modification, the parameters of which can be set in partnership with the GP or hospital consultant and delivered by the physiotherapists via a CMP with the agreement of the patient.

Exercise

Consider the range of conditions mentioned in this chapter and choose one which you might feel competent to prescribe for. Now access a CMP template on the Department of Health website and formulate one for a simulated patient using appropriate national and local guidelines as evidence. On completion make sure that you are aware of the pharmacological actions of all medicines included in the CMP, along with indications, contraindications, cautions, doses, formulations and drug interactions

Conclusion

The profession will continue to lobby for physiotherapists to gain independent prescribing rights as there are large groups of patients who present with acute musculoskeletal problems who would benefit from a physiotherapist

Conclusion cont'd

being able to prescribe. With the development of self-referral and direct referral into physiotherapy services and an active private sector where patients already self-refer plus the development of interface clinics, patients would benefit from more physiotherapists who can prescribe. This ability to prescribe as well as administer will enable patients to benefit from a truly 'one-stop' service for treatment of a range of conditions which include acute joint problems such as tennis elbow and soft tissue injuries including a range of sports injuries.

As independent prescribers physiotherapists would need to have access to a prescribing budget for patients within the NHS. For those outside the NHS the cost of prescribing can be passed on to the patient. The majority of independent prescribers are likely to be in the private sector where self-referral is widely practised. The main barrier in this sector would be private insurers many of whom see the GP or consultant as the referral route into physiotherapy.

As self-referral in the NHS develops, prescribing budgets will need to be developed either through acute NHS Trusts and PCTs or more generally through strategic health authorities.

As the profession of physiotherapy continues to develop, opportunities to improve the care given to patients will always be pursued by physiotherapists. Whereas in the past this was more likely to be in an informal manner with the need to provide evidence of efficacy and value for money, future advances are likely to be based on more research and an increasing evidence base. The desire to treat the patient holistically will continue.

Extending physiotherapy to include prescribing facilitates the holistic care of a patient combined with efficacy. This approach is likely to be cost-effective as it provides the patient with 'one-stop' care at the time required. This is an example of an extension to practice, which could be used as a model for future developments within the profession.

References

1. Chartered Society of Physiotherapy. *Curriculum Framework for Qualifying Physiotherapy Programs* (London: CSP, 2002).

2. Gardiner, J. and Wagstaff, S. 'Extended scope physiotherapy: The way towards consultant physiotherapists?' *Physiotherapy*, 87: 1 (2001) 2–3.

3. Department of Health. *The NHS Plan: A Plan for Investment, a Plan for Reform* (London: Crown Copyright, July 2000).

4. Department of Health and Social Security *Neighbourhood Nursing: A Focus for Care* (Cumberlege Report) (London: HMSO, 1986).

5. Department of Health. *Review of Prescribing, Supply and Administration of Medicines*, Final Report (Crown II) (London: DH, March 1999).

6. Department of Health. *Supplementary Prescribing by Nurses, Pharmacists, Chiropodists/Podiatrists, Physiotherapists and Radiographers within the NHS in England* (London: DH, 2005).

7. Statutory Instrument. The Medicines (Sale and Supply) (Miscellaneous Provisions) Amendment Regulations 2005.

Chapter 14
Podiatry and prescribing

Diane Birkinshaw

Introduction

Podiatry training entails a three-year degree course at a recognised university and consists of training in podiatry theory, anatomy, physiology, biomechanics, pathomechanics, pharmacology, medicine and research methods. This allows a practitioner to be registered with the Health Professions Council and to become a member of the Society of Podiatrists and Chiropodists. The pharmacology module results in a certificate in pharmacology and allows the podiatrist to supply and administer within the guidelines of PGDs. Now podiatrists can train as supplementary prescribers and work in partnerships with medical practitioners, prescribing treatments and medicines following the formulation of CMP for individual patients. Postgraduate courses are now available for podiatrists who wish to obtain this qualification. See Chapters 2, 3 and 18 for further information.

Podiatry Practice

The practice of podiatry has a wide remit from the reduction of callosities and treatment of nail pathologies such as ingrowing toe nails to the treatment of sports injuries and biomechanical assessments. The ability to prescribe pain relief for neuritis, along with treatments for bacterial and fungal infections, can only be beneficial. Most podiatrists working in the field of diabetes will find this a useful skill to enable them to manage care autonomously for the reasons discussed in this chapter.

Podiatry in the NHS has seen progressive changes since around 1990 particularly with regard to the management of the diabetic foot. The podiatrist has become an integral part of the multi-disciplinary team that cares for patients with diabetes and is often the first point of contact when a patient presents with an infected foot ulcer. Around 2 per cent of the UK population is believed to have diabetes of whom perhaps 200,000 have Type 1 diabetes and more than 1 million have Type 2 diabetes.[1] Foot ulceration is thought to affect 15 per cent of people with diabetes at some time in their lives.[2]

Foot Ulcers

The aetiology of diabetic foot ulcers can usually be attributed to one or a combination of the following factors:

- an impaired arterial supply
- neuropathy
- musculoskeletal deformities.

An ulcer is the result of a break in the dermal barrier of the skin often due to some form of trauma and once this has occurred the risk of infection is greatly increased. Infection will not necessarily cause an ulcer but it can increase the amount of damaged tissue. The management of these ulcers will include a variety of treatments, and patients often require antibiotics. It is imperative that infection is halted as this is a major contributory factor to amputation.[3]

Over recent years changes in the way patients can receive their medicines have progressed rapidly. The advent of supplementary prescribing to include podiatrists is likely to see many benefits in the management of patients with diabetic foot problems and hence diabetic services.[4]

Current Practice

The podiatrist who cares for the patient with diabetic foot ulcer will review the patient on a regular basis probably once or twice a week. The rationale for close supervision is that the problem can escalate rapidly in these patients as they may be immunocompromised or else insensitive to pain or deterioration of the wound due to peripheral neuropathy. Most patients will attend outpatient departments within hospital and GP settings. The podiatrist will undertake sharp debridement of callus and slough where necessary which is thought to be essential for optimizing healing rates.[5] This procedure involves the removal of callus or slough with a sharp instrument such as a surgical knife.

An assessment of the wound is made at each visit and includes the monitoring of wound exudate, surrounding skin condition, wound size, both depth and width, callus production and hence pressure relief. The podiatrist will also be monitoring the need to take wound swabs and check previous swab results and x-rays to assess infection status looking both for local infection and for osteomyelitis. The patient is holistically assessed in order to provide the most appropriate treatment with regard to wound healing and to obtain their agreement. Assessment of other factors including diabetes control, pain relief, referral for vascular procedures such as angiography and orthopaedic/orthotist referrals will also take place during the session.

Where there is no CMP in place and a patient requires antibiotics either on an initial basis or as a follow-up the podiatrist calls the 'on-call' diabetes team and requests a visit for the patient who will wait in the clinic until the doctor arrives. Once the doctor is available a consultation will take place to include the patient, podiatrist and the doctor. They will discuss what medication is required. This will usually be based on pathology, x-ray reports and clinical appearance of the wound and foot. The podiatrist indicates whether the wound is improving or deteriorating based on previous consultations and information from colleagues. Podiatrists work closely together in order to promote collaborative working and continuity of care.

At times it is not possible to contact on-call teams and patients are not always able to wait for the doctor. In these instances the GP is contacted for a prescription. Although GPs are very responsive to requests, this practice does cause delays to patient therapy and creates extra work for the podiatrist. They not only have to make telephone contact but several practices also require fax requests.

The patient is usually allocated a half-hour appointment for treatment but as can be seen, these appointments often become protracted due to the patients having to wait for doctors who are otherwise busy. Time is an issue for both clinician and patient for a variety of reasons. For the clinician, the workload is ever increasing and there are a vast number of patients with foot ulcers. For the patient, many have jobs to attend or other activities they would rather be doing and can get frustrated with numerous appointments and time delays.

Prescriptions for dressings also need to be considered and this has often required the podiatrist to make contact with a practice nurse or district nurse to prescribe the appropriate dressings. This can only take place once the nurse has assessed the patient them-selves. This again is time-consuming as well as causing a delay in patient care, as podiatrists are unable to access certain prescription-only dressings and patients therefore have to wait for these to become available. With the advent of silver dressings and other prescription-only dressings this practice of phoning for prescriptions is ever increasing.

The Future

Supplementary prescribing for podiatrists within the remit of treating patients with diabetic foot problems appears to bring with it many advantages not only for the practitioners but also for the patients. Time delays caused by the need to contact other health care professionals to process prescriptions could potentially be reduced and the need for patients to be sitting around waiting for doctors eliminated. Often antibiotics need to be administered on that day to avoid the risk of increasing infection, hospital admission and possible amputation.

Case study

A gentleman attends with a neuropathic foot ulcer on the plantar aspect of the first metatarsal which is infected with pseudomonas bacteria. He experiences pain in the feet from neuritis due to poor diabetes control. As these types of infection can be anticipated, CMPs can be agreed with the consultant diabetologist and patient, for a six-week course of antibiotics, a treatment for painful peripheral neuropathy and a silver-containing dressing, all of which could be prescribed by the podiatrist. These then could be re-prescribed as necessary by the podiatrist rather than the doctor or nurse.

Exercise

Consider the scenario above and access a blank CMP template on the Department of Health website. Formulate a CMP for the condition and use national and local guidelines to support it. Ensure that you know the pharmacology of the medicines included, along with indications, contraindications, cautions, dose, side effects, formulations and possible drug interactions. Consider co-morbidities in relation to such prescribing.

During the podiatry consultation the patient often builds a rapport with the clinician which increases their confidence in the decisions that are being made for the treatment of their foot. This occurs due to the frequency and length of appointments. However, as seen in nursing there is a definite lack of public knowledge which could be transcribed to podiatry where there is an ignorance of their skills.[6] In view of this it is necessary to educate the patients regarding prescribing skills of podiatrists. This is likely to be driven by opportunistic education for patients, team work within the multi-disciplinary setting and support of the governing body, the Society of Podiatrists and Chiropodists and the NHS management teams. Team working amongst agencies is paramount and should encourage the break down of professional boundaries which can occur when clinicians take on the existing roles of others. The podiatrist needs to know that the patient is confident with the decisions they are making for their care and see them as specialists who are able to take on new roles.[7]

It can, however, often be seen that patients feel more comfortable when seeing a clinician they know well rather than a doctor who is not familiar with their foot condition. This happens when a junior member of the diabetes team is called and the patient will not disclose certain information and often appears happier to share information regarding levels of pain and compliance with the podiatrist. The podiatrist is dealing with wounds on a daily basis and so they have enormous experience with regard to wound healing and infection.

Supplementary prescribing will encourage autonomy for podiatrists which could be both a motivator and confidence booster particularly if they see it as making their work schedules more effective. However, there will still be a need to work within a team perhaps more so in order to ensure that continuity of care is not compromised. Working together to develop PGDs can result in energising people and result in new ways of tackling old problems.[8] This can relate to podiatrists working within the NHS but not those in the private sector who do not have access to PGDs and are looking for other ways notably through an exemption order to access antibiotics, analgesics, treatments for fungal infection and dressings.

Podiatrists are used to working independently and making diagnoses; however, those working in the field of diabetes and other chronic diseases such as rheumatoid arthritis are used to working collaboratively in a multi-disciplinary team where it is essential for the clinician to have excellent communication skills.

Current methods of note-taking need to be addressed with the advent of supplementary prescribing. There needs to be shared access to notes in order that the podiatrist has all the information required to fulfil total patient care. This involves improvement with computer systems so that audit can also be carried out. Other issues to address are those of budgets, for both prescribing and education. The need for good mentors and sufficient education programmes would have to be considered which does, however, place stress on existing work loads of clinicians.

Conclusion

Supplementary prescribing would appear to be the way forward for podiatrists working in the field of diabetology, rheumatology and with musculoskeletal conditions, particularly for those clinicians who become consultant podiatrists. With good collaborative practice and the ironing out of any logistical problems the service users would all benefit from this forward-thinking practice.

References

1. Calman, K. *On the State of the Public Health.* The Annual Report of the Chief Medical Officer of The Department of Health For The Year 1997 (London: The Stationary Office, 1998).

2. Spencer, S. 'Pressure relieving interventions for preventing and treating diabetic foot ulcers' (Cochrane Review). In: *The Cochrane Library,* Update Software, Oxford. Issue 4 (2000).

3. Reiber, G., Pecoraro, R. and Koepsell, T. 'Risk factors for amputation in patients with diabetes mellitus: A case control study'. *Annals of Internal Medicine,* 117 (1992) 97–105.

4. Kerr, D. and Allen, D. 'The diabetic foot at the crossroads: vanguard or oblivion?' *The Diabetic Foot,* 3:3 (2000) 70–74.

5. Edmonds, M. and Foster, A. *Managing Stage 3: The Ulcerated Foot.* In: Edmonds, M. and Foster, A. *Managing the Diabetic Foot.* (London: Blackwell Science, 2000).

6. Furlong, S. and Glover, D. 'Confusion surrounds piecemeal changes in nurse's roles'. *Nursing Times*, 94:37 (1998) 54–56.

7. Mckenna, H. and Keeney, S. 'Community nursing: Health professional and public perceptions'. *Journal of Advanced Nursing*, 48:1 (2004) 17–25.

8. Davies, C. 'Getting health professional to work together'. *British Medical Journal*, 320 (2000) 1021–1022.

Chapter 15

Radiography and prescribing

Josie Cameron

Introduction

The role of the radiographer has evolved over the years, directed by the need for highly skilled professionals to extend their role in order to benefit patients. In some instances this has arisen as a direct result of a more flexible approach to multi-disciplinary team working and skill mix within departments of clinical oncology.[1] Responsibilities previously in the domain of doctors have now become a routine part of the role of suitably experienced and qualified radiographers. Examples of this include:

- gaining consent to radiotherapy treatment
- radiographer-led simulation +/− computerised tomography (CT) planning
- supply and administration of palliative treatment under PGDs
- on treatment review clinics, follow-up clinics
- brachytherapy.

Therapy radiographers are part of an oncology team that treat patients who have cancer.[2] They utilise ionising radiation in the form of high energy x-rays to accurately deliver a radiation dose to the site of the cancer whilst minimising exposure to normal, healthy tissue. A therapy radiographer is involved in every aspect of treatment including pre-treatment preparation, planning, the treatment itself and the review or follow-up stages.[2] As a result of the diversity of the role, it is essential that radiographers have excellent interpersonal skills to communicate with other members of the team and also to provide support and information to patients and their carers. Extensive knowledge of cancer and its management is mandatory, and it is interesting to note that therapy radiographers are the only health care professionals whose sole training is in oncology and the treatment of cancer. Not only team working but also the ability to work independently are requirements, as is the ability to learn new skills and adapt to the continually changing technological environment.

New responsibilities allow radiographers to utilise existing experience and gain new skills and knowledge whilst freeing up valuable medical time.[3] It is therefore cost-effective and an efficient use of resources which should not compromise patient care or safety.

Another area where radiographers are becoming increasingly involved is in the supply or administration of medications to patients under a PGD. One of the main benefits of a PGD is that it gives the patient quick access to the appropriate medication for treatment-related toxicities. As a result the PGD has become a successful tool in oncology practice as patients are able to receive specified creams or medications without a medical consultation. Another benefit of a PGD is that it may help address issues surrounding evidence-based care and/or adherence to local and national guidelines regarding the medication to be supplied or administered as a result of the specific inclusion criteria[4] required (see Chapter 18 for more information regarding PGDs).

Supplementary Prescribing

Supplementary prescribing is a natural progression from the use of PGDs, currently utilised by many radiographers. It allows radiographers to assess individual patients and prescribe medication using a patient-specific CMP in partnership with an independent prescriber who will be a doctor. In effect the benefit to patients will be great as an immediate decision can be made regarding the patient's condition and the most appropriate medication can be prescribed, as long as it is included in the CMP, thus avoiding any delays.

Treatment toxicity varies for different treatment sites and is influenced by the effect of prior or concomitant chemotherapy; therefore the medication to be prescribed may in fact be necessary as a result of the chemotherapy-induced reaction and not just from the radiotherapy. Treatment review clinics offer the most appropriate way of assessing the patient as well as offering support and advice when patients are suffering from a treatment-related problem. It may also be necessary to check for concordance with the medications prescribed as many patients do not adhere to the advice given to them. The reasons for this may be multi-factorial and it is important for the radiographer to help the patient to gain the required benefit from their medications.

The group of patients most likely to benefit from this innovative role extension are those suffering from head and neck cancer as they suffer the most treatment-related toxicity. Oral mucosa is extremely sensitive to radiotherapy and oro-pharyngeal mucositis may be the major treatment dose-limiting factor in this cohort of patients. It is estimated that approximately 15 per cent of patients treated with radical radiotherapy to the oral cavity or pharynx will require hospitalisation for treatment-related complications.[5]

The addition of concomitant chemotherapy may cause a more severe breakdown of the mucosa and the skin within the irradiated area, which in turn causes the patient a great deal of discomfort and pain. These patients need a lot of support throughout their treatment and constant monitoring of their medications to minimise their distress. The supplementary prescribing radiographer would be ideally placed to review such patients and the patients would benefit as they would not be limited to one medical consultation per week as radiographers could be more flexible in their consultations.

Acute skin reactions are the most frequently occurring side effect of radiation; published reports suggest that 90–95 per cent of patients experience some degree of reaction.[6] Therefore, skin-related toxicity can be a problem for all sites irradiated and medications to prevent or heal desquamation reactions are commonplace. Minor infections post surgery are also common and patients often present with typical symptoms of erythema, heat and inflammation which used to necessitate a consultation with a doctor.

Radiographers have vast experience of skin reactions as they see the patients on a daily basis and are therefore ideally placed to recognise any unusual skin discolouration and to take appropriate action.

Many patients with breast cancer are routinely prescribed hormonal medications such as tamoxifen as an adjuvant form of treatment which can be taken at the same time as their radiotherapy. These hormonal treatments induce an artificial menopausal effect on the patient causing them to suffer from hot flushes, night sweats, vaginal discharge and dryness which can be quite detrimental to the patient's quality of life.[7] Younger women suffer more severe side effects related to the loss of reproductive function plus more abrupt vaginal changes than older women as a result of an artificially induced menopause.[8] The review radiographer trained in supplementary prescribing would be able to determine the severity of these side effects during the consultation and prescribe an appropriate medication via a CMP to help alleviate these distressing symptoms.

Another benefit to patients would be in prescribing the hormonal treatment as poor communication between hospital staff and the GP can mean that patients are not receiving their prescriptions at the appropriate time. This obviously delays the start of the hormonal treatment and may cause the patient to be concerned and anxious regarding any potential detrimental effect.

The Society of Radiographers has strong views on prescribing and its vision statement, 'radiographer prescribing is not an option for the future, it is a requirement', serves to highlight its stance.[9] Supplementary prescribing therefore will benefit the profession by recognising the existing skills and experience that radiographers possess, it will allow for the development of new responsibilities (with training and supervision) and, as a result of this role extension, may allow for further career progression, for example consultant radiographer posts. Radiographers are likely to embrace this new concept and view this as a unique opportunity to advance the profession and, as a result, improve the service to patients.

Patients will benefit as a result of prompt and efficient service, reduced delays in the decision-making process and completion of the prescription where necessary along with increased continuity of care. New closer working relationships will also be forged between the independent prescriber and the supplementary prescriber, which should benefit both the patient and the workplace.

There remains potential for problems to arise, however, as a result of this new role. Some doctors may feel their territory is being invaded and may view this crossing of role boundaries in a negative light. It may also be perceived as threatening to the role of the junior doctor/registrar as their place in the hierarchy may be altered, but the main issue is it challenges the accepted role and responsibilities of the radiographer as viewed by the medical profession.

Exercise

The response by the doctor's professional bodies to the expansion of prescribing rights to the non-medical professions has been less than enthusiastic. Some of their concerns relate to some of the issues discussed above. How would you defend the role of the radiographer as a supplementary prescriber?

Other potential problems include:

- time-consuming study away from the workplace, approximately 38 days
- cost of the course may be prohibitive if self-funded
- availability of mentors to facilitate learning and provide supervision.

These problems may be alleviated by e-learning and distance learning provision and by departmental funding of places on the required training programmes.

Future Developments

With the advent of the new consultant radiographer role and the opportunity for role extension and responsibilities, it will be essential to expand prescribing rights to that of an independent prescriber. The consultant radiographers will have their own workload and will be responsible for the patients in their care, including assessment and diagnosis of treatment-related morbidities. It would seem sensible to aim for independent prescribing once supplementary prescribing has been in operation and suitable training has been established. The curriculum for the training programme for certain AHPs to train as supplementary prescribers has already been prepared and has recently been approved by the Department of Health. It provides a positive commitment to role extension of AHPs and identifies the training needs of this staff group, and addresses critical issues such as competency.[10]

Conclusion

The many positive benefits of supplementary prescribing rights for radiographers far outweigh the potential problems that may arise and should not hinder the progress of this new role development.

For supplementary and independent prescribing to succeed it requires progressive, forward-thinking doctors to 'lead' and develop the partnership. This should help to ensure that the transition radiographers will undertake in order to become supplementary prescribers is a smooth one.

Radiographers will require supervision and support especially in the early stages but ultimately the outcome should ensure an equal, working partnership between doctor, radiographer and the patient. It is also important to note that once sufficient numbers of AHPs have become experienced in their role, they may be able to act as mentors to other trainee supplementary prescribers relieving the burden from already overstretched medical staff. Presently only doctors can be mentors for non-medical prescribers but this may change in the future.

References

1. The Royal College of Radiologists. *Breaking the Mould: Roles, Responsibilities and Skills Mix in Departments of Clinical Oncology* (London: Intertype, 2002).

2. The Society of Radiographers Website. *Careers Information.* www.sor.org, accessed 02/05/05.

3. National Prescribing Centre. *Supplementary Prescribing: A Resource to help Healthcare Professionals to Understand the Framework and Opportunities.* (NPC: April 2003).

4. Flint, H. 'Patient group directions in an oncology setting'. *Pharmacy Management*, 18: 3 (2002) 39–43.

5. Peters, L., Ang, K. and Thames, H. *Altered Fractionation Schedules.* In: Perez, C. and Brady, L. (eds) *Principles and Practice of Radiation Oncology* (Philadelphia: JB Lippincott, 1992) 97–113.

6. Porock, D. and Kristjanson, L. 'Skin reactions during radiotherapy for breast cancer: The use and impact of topical agents and dressings'. *European Journal of Cancer Care*, 8 (1999) pp. 144–153.

7. Daly, E., Gray, A., Barlow, D., McPherson, K., Roche, M. and Vessey, M. 'Measuring the impact of menopausal symptoms on quality of life'. *British Medical Journal*, 307 (1993) pp. 836–840.

8. Stead, M. 'Sexual dysfunction after treatment for gynaecologic and breast malignancies'. *Current Opinion in Obstetric Gynaecology*, 15: 1 (2003) pp. 57–61.

9. The Society and College of Radiographers. *Prescribing by Radiographers: A Vision Paper by the College of Radiographers* (London: Society and College of Radiographers, 2001).

10. Department of Health. *Outline Curriculum for Training Programmes to Prepare Allied Health Professionals as Supplementary Prescribers* (September 2004). www.dh.gov.uk/assetRoot/01/08/90/03/04089003.pdf, accessed 12/05/05.

Part IV

Developments in Practice

Chapter 16

Implementing prescribing in secondary care

Ruth Oliver-Williams

Introduction

Historically only medical staff have had the ability to prescribe both in the primary and secondary care settings, however, with the advent of non-medical prescribing a multi-professional workforce now has the ability to contribute to the therapeutic management of patient care.

This chapter will give an overview of how one Acute NHS Trust in England introduced non-medical prescribing into the secondary care environment, the benefits and the challenges. This account relates to practice that was constrained by the extended formulary for nurses. It commences with a detailed account of the assessment and analysis of the personnel and culture, followed by the approach taken to introduce this new concept into the clinical environment.

The historical role of the nurse in medicines management has revolved around the safe administration of prescribed medication to patients. Through effective communication channels with medical colleagues, nurses have played a pivotal role in ensuring that prescribed treatments meet with the needs of patients. Until recent years, however, they were powerless to plan and prescribe treatments themselves. Nurses' professional skills and judgement have previously been underutilised in the field of medicines management, yet it now realised the positive contribution that nurse prescribing has on patient care.[1] The current mechanisms available for the prescribing, supply and administration of medicines to the general public in the secondary care sector are:

- PSDs
- PGDs

189

▶ independent nurse prescribing (soon to include independent pharmacist prescribing)
▶ supplementary prescribing
▶ Specific exemptions covering supply or administration by certain professionals, for example midwives as contained in medicines legislation.[2]

At the time of writing hospitals in the United Kingdom have small numbers of nurse prescribers partly due to the ongoing use of PGDs and partly as a result of the medical dominance in the management of patient caseloads. It was the aim of the current government to train several hundred pharmacists to become supplementary prescribers and several thousand nurses to become extended and supplementary prescribers by the end of 2004. The situation has now moved on. Nurses and pharmacists now perform as independent prescribers, mainly due to the very good evaluation of the performance of these professions within their previously limited roles. This allows for improved patient access to medicines, enhanced skills of nurses and pharmacists, therefore resulting in an improved NHS. The need to reduce junior doctors' hours coupled with the effect of the new foundation training for junior grade medical staff and a large percentage of GPs opting out of 'out of hours' services has left a huge demand for continuity in the management of patients with LTCs. Nurses and pharmacists, along with other AHPs are already bringing their expertise into this area and prescribing will be and already is very much a part of this shift in responsibility.

Change Management

Within the current climate of health care delivery there are many pressures and constraints to providing a comprehensive and evidence-based service. There has been a drive from the Department of Health and professional bodies to continuously monitor practice and make the appropriate changes to service delivery[3] to ensure that standards of care are safe, measurable and appropriate to the situation. Change management theory provides some useful instruction about the introduction of new ways of working or the requirement to adapt current practice. Prior to introducing change into an area, an overview of the organisational culture including exploring stakeholder interests and barriers to implementing the change must be examined to identify any key areas of concern.[4] The culture of an organisation can have a profound effect on the adoption of new initiatives, how it affects the way in which things are done, how people are treated and how it will influence people's ideas of what they are there for.[4,5] It is important to identify driving and restraining forces when introducing change. It has been proposed that assessment of the forces will identify the constraints and barriers to the introduction of a new initiative and will underline the likely commitment of the stakeholders, internal and external to the organisation. This activity may also act as an indicator of the time and effort required to implement a change and it may also predict the degree of success.[4] In order to identify and analyse the environment within the hospital Trust a PESTEL analysis[4] and a force field analysis[6] were completed to help determine key areas of concern and to highlight the potential driving and restraining forces. See Tables 16.1 and 16.2. The PESTEL analysis is a useful tool for determining factors that are either proving helpful or impeding progress but it also has its critics. As with any tool it is its application to the situation that is key. It can become a paper exercise that highlights the issues but does not consider how they may be addressed. It has similarities with Lewin's force field analysis as the driving and restraining forces are represented by the 'helpful' and 'impeding' factors identified. Lewin[6] suggested that by reducing restraining forces, one allows the natural progression of driving forces to introduce the change.

Exercise

Examine the reference texts given here to become more familiar with these models and theories. Consider the change in prescribing practice in your area. Is it popular and is it sustained? What are the determining factors?

Additionally it has been suggested by many authors that different styles of organisational cultures exist[25,26,27] and these need to be considered when introducing change into any work environment.

In order to introduce the change it was necessary to explore practices by investigating views relating to non-medical prescribing within specific staff groups in the organisation. It was already known that only three nursing staff possessed an extended prescribing qualification and that there were emerging needs from

Table 16.1 PESTEL analysis

	Helpful factors	Factors likely to impede progress
Political	The Crown Report[7] Nurse Prescribers' Formulary[8] Making a Difference[9] Section 63, Health & Social Care Act [10] The NHS Plan, Department of Health[11] Department of Health & Medicines Control Agency public consultation April–July[12] Commission for Health Improvement Reduction in junior doctors' hours and the European Working Time Directive Reforming emergency care strategy[13]	Doctors' lack of knowledge of developments Public perceptions Nurses' inability to adopt the role due to scepticism Organisations' difficulty in accepting the benefits and providing the infrastructure
Economic	Actual cost of increased length of stay Prescribing budget	Financial constraints of NHS budget PCT commissioning budget
Social	Improved patient journey and outcomes related to quality of care Improved job satisfaction for nurses and pharmacists	Perceived erosion of medical roles Lack of incentives for nurses, pharmacists and AHPs to train
Technological	Agenda for Change knowledge and skills framework[14]	Limitations of electronic communication systems across secondary and primary care Lack of IT literacy amongst staff Slow implementation of NHS IT strategy
Ecological	Patients' expectation that the 'most appropriate care will be delivered by the most skilled manpower, and by the best able to deliver it'	An environment that lacks adequate support for this role A culture that is unaccepting of nurses extending their responsibilities

Legal (Medico-legal)	Health & Social Care Act[10] Amendments to the Prescription Only Medicines Order[15] Changes to NHS regulations NMC Scope of Professional Practice[16] NMC Code of Professional Conduct: standards for conduct, performance and ethics[17] NMC Guidelines for records and record keeping[18] NMC Covert administration of medicines[19] Fitness to practice[20] Fitness to practice and purpose[21] NMC Guidelines for the administration of medicines[22] NMC circular 25-2002 Independent and supplementary prescribing[23]	Chapter six prescriptions and requisitions www.the-shipman-inquiry.org.uk/fourthreport.asp[24] Lack of awareness of the legal implications of prescribing mistakes. Doctors' reticence at entering a partnership with nurse and patient to develop CMPs Preference to continue using PGDs

Table 16.2 Force field analysis

Forces driving change	Restraining forces
Local, regional and national policy initiatives (National Service frameworks; NHS Plan) Clinical governance/higher education institutions resource management Patient/client needs → Cost reduction pressures → DOH targets →	Local inertia from within the Trust Tradition of medical dominance, fear of change ← Budgetary constraints

many of the departments to equip their staff with new skills and knowledge to benefit patient care. What was not known was the reason for the small numbers of prescribers. Were staff reluctant to undertake the training or were the mechanisms not in place to facilitate their support in carrying out the training? An audit of pharmacists, specialist nurses and emergency nurse practitioners was undertaken to ascertain their understanding and desire to undertake a prescribing course. A set of eight questions was distributed through the hospital e-mail system to selected personnel. This audit determined that a core group of individuals were interested in adding a prescribing qualification to their day-to-day practice. A number of both nurses and pharmacists expressed an interest in enrolling on the next available course.

Eligibility criteria was devised following guidance set by the Department of Health and NMC; they closely reflected the needs of the organisation, local development plans and patient needs. Interested individuals were then invited to apply to a university of their choice to commence their prescribing training. Alongside this a competency tool was adapted from the National Prescribing Centre allowing management to safely support and facilitate each 'student prescriber' in attaining competency in his or her new role.

One issue the Trust faced was how it would meet the ongoing professional development needs of the new prescribers? With the educational resources being tied to specific universities it was difficult to plan how to meet the needs of a diverse group of individuals without additional funding. A suggestion was made to the SHA that resources and knowledge be shared to tackle the issue. This was not felt to be a priority at that time, hence the Trust was still unaware of how to provide highly specialised education, maintaining the competency of new prescribers in practice. See Chapter 19 for discussions on maintaining competency in prescribing.

Another aspect of non-medical prescribing training is the need for the student to have a medical mentor to assess practice. The secondary care staff that had chosen to undertake the prescribing course found that the medical facilitators approached were willing to be involved in their training. This has not been the case for some colleagues in primary care who have struggled to find medical facilitators amongst GPs.

'A structured logical approach' was adopted to introduce non-medical prescribing into the Trust, a project plan was devised with an associated timeline and outcome measures. Each outcome was assigned to an individual or a team and the timescales set were adjustable and achievable. See Table 16.3.

At the time of writing 8 nurses and 2 pharmacists had applied to commence the relevant prescribing courses, at various centres in the South East of England. Currently, one nurse and one pharmacist have successfully completed the supplementary prescribing course and are now practicing as supplementary prescribers in the care of patients with LTCs in the acute setting.

Table 16.3 Project plan

Objective	Action	Review	Completed
Identify practitioners willing to undertake the course	Questionnaire to specialist nurses, pharmacists and emergency nurse practitioners	One month	Yes. August 2004
Ascertain availability of suitable prescribing courses within the SHA meeting Trust needs	Speak to commissioning manager and finance manager SHA	Two months	Yes – November 2004
Identify available courses and suitable medical mentors	Liaise with Trust Medical Director and Clinical Directors. Collate register of medical mentors	Ongoing	Yes, but ongoing item
Initiate a web-based resource containing relevant information regarding prescribing	Initiate contact with Trust webmaster and the IT department	Six months	Yes, but ongoing item
Investigate ongoing CPD needs of potential extended and supplementary prescribers within the Trust	Liaise with Assistant Director of Practice Development and Head of Education and Training (Organisational Development)	Six monthly/ annually	Yes, but ongoing item
Devise an audit process for the yellow card scheme	Discuss with clinical audit and pharmacy	6–8 months	No ongoing
Collate a list of local and national guidelines Investigate PRODIGY	Communicate with the medicines usage committee and the chief pharmacist	Ongoing	Ongoing
Examine potential compatibility of patient record systems	Discuss needs with Integrated Care Record Scheme (ICRS) project manager. Review regularly	Ongoing – dynamic item	Ongoing due to postponement of ICRS

Table 16.3 (Continued)

Objective	Action	Review	Completed
Disseminating information relating to the role of the extended and supplementary prescriber and the application to practice	Discuss with Assistant Director Practice Development and Chief pharmacist	Ongoing	Ongoing
Examine legal and professional implications including vicarious liability	Discuss with Director of Nursing implications of extended and supplementary prescribing in the clinical environment	3 months	Completed – November 2004
Establish format for supervised practice and ongoing support mechanisms within the Trust	Discuss with Assistant Director, Practice Development, and Medical Director	6 months	Ongoing.

Exercise

How many non-medical prescribers are there in your area of work? Reflect on the culture of your organisation and whether non-medical prescribing would benefit patient care. How could this be further enhanced by supplementary prescribing for AHPs and independent and supplementary prescribing for nurses and pharmacists? Can you devise a proposal to support your answers to these questions?

Nurse Independent Prescribing in Secondary Care

Nurse prescribing is invaluable for emergency nurse practitioners working in the minor injuries department. This facility enables them to diagnose, treat and discharge patients with minor sprains and muscular injuries without having to ask a doctor for prescriptions for simple analgesia, as well improving the service for patients complaining of minor aches and pains. Previously, many senior nurses voiced the need to expand their skills to encompass an aspect of prescribing, they did not feel the need to undertake the training programme as they felt that PSDs and PGDs usually met their needs. There is an argument that sometimes PGDs have been used beyond their remit and this is discussed in more detail in Chapter 18. Emergency nurse practitioners have found prescribing directly for patients has worked to their advantage. The role has allowed them to expedite patient waiting times for treatments giving them increased job satisfaction whilst providing a better service for patients.

Views of a Nurse Prescriber

What follows are the views of nurse prescriber for undertaking nurse prescribing:

> 'the main reason for undertaking the nurse prescribing course was to be able to complete an episode of care for patients. Within the Minor Injuries Unit (MIU), I would see, treat and discharge patients independently until they needed medication. I would then have to ask the doctor for the prescription. This could sometimes mean a lengthy wait and most doctors, quite rightly, would like to see the patient themselves before prescribing. This again caused delays for patients and duplication of work. I also felt that having to ask for a prescription undermined my role as a nurse practitioner. This was particularly frustrating when the doctor I would refer to told me I had more experience in dealing with minor injuries than he did!'

Supplementary Prescribing

Supplementary prescribing partnerships will continue to be utilised by nurses and pharmacists in some instances and by AHPs in all instances in relation to prescribing appropriately for patients in their care.

The partnership between the independent prescriber (doctor or dentist) and supplementary prescriber is of paramount importance. Roles and responsibilities need to be identified clearly. This should be facilitated by effective communication, resulting in safe and effective prescribing for patients. The prescribing partners have responsibility to ensure that the criterion for lawful supplementary prescribing is maintained. See Chapters 2, 3 and 18 for more detail.

Supplementary prescribers utilise CMPs in practice to manage an individual patient's treatment regime. Within individual organisations there may be discussions between the medical director, clinical colleagues and general managers to ascertain which conditions supplementary prescribers may prescribe for, within the remits of their role. In this Trust each student prescriber was asked to develop a list of CMP templates to be validated by the clinical effectiveness committee for use in his or her practice. These would be later individualised to treat appropriate patients.

Exercise

This chapter has discussed the issues of changing practice in the acute setting, particularly in respect of the role of the specialist nurse. Identify other professionals involved in caring for in-patients or in out-patient clinics who may benefit from extending their roles to encompass a prescribing remit.

You may identify the pharmacist, physiotherapist or chiropodist/podiatrist. Interview one of these professionals about their perception of this.

Other chapters in this book are written by these professionals. Compare their views with those of the people you have spoken to.

Conclusion

Non-medical prescribing offers each patient comprehensive and continuous management of their condition(s) by suitably qualified health care professionals. The ability to prescribe for acute and long-term conditions gives clinical credibility and greater job satisfaction to health professionals that undertake the role. Health professionals are likely to develop better relationships with patients, imparting specialist knowledge and preparing them to manage their condition in consultation with the health professional seeing them on a regular basis.

Often in current practice the patient is left out of the decision-making process.[28] There may be a discrepancy between the doctor's and patient's perception regarding the impact of a disease.[29] There is a need for holistic prescribing to improve the patient's experience and the impact of a condition on their day-to-day lives. The advent of non-medical prescribing will help to address some of these issues.

The extension of non-medical prescribing rights is therefore to be welcomed. The argument supporting this development particularly from the primary care perspective has been explored elsewhere within this text. This chapter has focused on developing the role in the acute sector. Within secondary care it is a positive step that will be embraced enthusiastically by specialist nurses and will be a bonus in the re-configuration of service delivery.

References

1. Humphries, J. and Green, J. (eds). *Nurse Prescribing* (Basingstoke: Macmillan, 1999).

2. Modernisation Agency. *Medicines Matters: A Guide to Current Mechanisms for the Prescribing, Supply and Administration of Medicines* (London: DH, 2005) p. 24.

3. Carlopio, J., Andrewartha, G. and Armstrong, H. *Developing Management Skills in Australia.* 1st edition (Sydney: Longman, 1997).

4. Critical Appraisal Skills Programme (CASP) *Evidence Based Healthcare: An Open Resource for Healthcare Practitioners* (Luton: Chiltern Press, 1999).

5. Iles, V. and Sutherland, K. *Organisational Change: A Review for Healthcare Managers, Professionals and Researchers.* National Coordinating Centre for NHS Service Delivery and Organisation R&D: 104 (2001).

6. Lewin, K. *Field Theory in Social Science* (London: Harper, 1951).

7. DH. *Review of Prescribing, Supply and Administration of Medicines. A Report on the Supply and Administrations of Medicines under Group Protocols* (Crown Report) (London: DH, 1998).

8. DH. *Nurse Prescribers Formulary* (London: DH, 1994).

9. DH. *Making a Difference* (London: DH, 2001).

10. DH. *Health & Social Care Act* (London: DH, 2001).

11. DH. *The NHS Plan* (London: DH, 2000).

12. Department of Health & Medicines Control Agency. *Public Consultation April–July* (London: DH, 2002).

13. DH. *Reforming Emergency Care Strategy* (London: DH, 2001).

14. DH. *Agenda for Change Knowledge and Skills Framework* (London: DH, 2003).

15. DH. *Amendment to the Prescription Only Medicines (POM) Order* (London: DH, 2001).

16. NMC. *Scope of Professional Practice* (London: NMC, 2002).

17. NMC. *The Code of Professional Conduct: Standards for Conduct, Performance and Ethics* (London: NMC, 2004).

18. NMC. *Guideline for Records and Record Keeping* (London: NMC, 2004).

19. NMC. *Covert Administration of Medicines* (London: NMC, 2001).

20. NMC. *Fitness for Practice* (London: NMC, 1999).

21. NMC. *Fitness for Practice and Purpose* (London: NMC, 2001).

22. NMC. *Guidelines for the Administration of Medicines* (London: NMC, 2004).

23. NMC. *Circular 25, Independent and Supplementary Prescribing* (London: NMC, 2002).

24. Chapter six. *Prescriptions and Requisitions.* www.the-shipman-inquiry.org.uk/fourthreport.asp, accessed 04/07/05.

25. Binney, G. and Williams, C. *Leaning into the Future: Changing the Way People Change Organisations* (London: Nicholas Brealey Publishing, 1997).

26. Handy, C. *Beyond Certainty: The Changing Worlds of Organisations* (London: Hutchinson, 1995).

27. Handy, C. *Understanding Organisations* (London: Penguin Business, 1993).

28. Oliver-Williams, R. *A Phenomenological Exploration of Chronic Obstructive Pulmonary Disease (COPD). What are the Experiences of Living with COPD? The Patient's perspective. Unpublished Thesis* (University of Oxford, 2004).

29. Dekhuijzen, P. 'The confronting COPD International survey: Patients hardly know they have COPD'. *European Respiratory Journal*, 20 (2002) 793–794.

Chapter 17

Prescribing in nurse triage situations

Sue Garratt

Introduction

The development of nurse-led triage services in primary care is becoming more popular.[1,2] The role of nurses in screening and treating patients presenting with undifferentiated, undiagnosed conditions and minor illnesses has underpinned new models of 'one-stop shops', exemplified by NHS Direct in England, NHS24 in Scotland and Primary Care Walk-in Centres (see Chapter 5). In order to provide a seamless consultation for the patient, the introduction of non-medical prescribing has been of major benefit in this area of primary care, allowing nurses to provide and complete a consultation. This improves patients' access to health care professionals, and, more specifically, enables them to see the health care professional most appropriate to their needs at the time.

Triage systems have been shown to help in reducing GP home visits by up to 50 per cent[3] and GP appointments by 40 per cent.[1] This chapter will be focusing on the uses of prescribing in nurse triage and will consider both telephone and face-to-face settings.

Nurse Telephone Triage

Nurse telephone triage has been present in various health care settings for a number of years, originating in secondary care where it was used predominantly in accident and emergency (A&E) departments.[4,5] In primary care it can actively assist in reducing or reorganising workloads when planned and implemented carefully, using experienced nursing staff.

Telephone triage gives patients an alternative point of access to the health system. What matters most to people is being able to access the health service speedily and effectively when they need it. Developments in primary care over the past few years have provided opportunities to review the skills of all disciplines and use them in new and innovative ways. The traditional role of the GP as 'gatekeeper' to the health system is being challenged by offering alternative routes for patients to obtain advice and treatments.[6]

The provision of information and support through triage may better inform patients about their health, public health matters, choices and treatments for illnesses. Isolated communities with poor transport, for example in farming areas, or patients who are not registered with a GP such as travellers or asylum seekers may benefit from the more flexible approach offered by these systems. Where patients present with problems that are outside the competence of the nurse such as mental health problems they would be referred to see a GP.

Exercise

Reflect on an instance when you might choose to seek advice via this method.

Analyse the barriers to communication that you could have encountered as a service user

Telephone consultation is not an exact science, and decision-making on the telephone differs vastly from critical thinking in a face-to-face consultation. There are several different models of telephone consultation[7] as shown in Table 17.1.

Of the three models mentioned in Table 17.1, studies have found that the guideline approach is most favoured by nurses and doctors and provides safer more effective outcomes.[3,8]

Exercise

Choose one of the telephone consultation methods and try it out with a colleague. Use a common complaint that a patient might call with and write down how you structured the consultation, the differential diagnoses made, your final diagnosis and any treatment or advice given as a result of the consultation.

Table 17.1   Models used in telephone consultations

Guideline approach	Structured assessment, with suggested questions, and decision paths in response to data input in answer to the previous questions. This approach allows the questions to be viewed before selection and movement between different assessment guidelines. The user is able to build up a profile of the patient.
The Protocol approach	A rigid pathway for assessment, allowing little or no direction by the user to determine the pathway. Once a pathway is selected, the pathway is pre-determined. Often previous questions are hidden, preventing the use of the 'whole picture' of a patient.
Binary Algorithm approach	Similar to the protocol approach, but the responses are 'yes' or 'no' to specific questions. The user has no discretion in selecting or answering questions. The answer determines the pathway down a decision tree. An algorithm has to be selected early in the consultation and answers have to be given to all questions, which can lead to lengthy consultation times.

All aspects of nursing expertise are used within a telephone triage consultation and all are important aspects to consider when prescribing. Effective listening skills and a non-judgmental attitude are essential to help develop a therapeutic relationship with the patient.

Some triage systems, for example Telephone Advice Software (TAS), use computerised protocols which may link to a prescribing decision; however, this does not allow triage nurses to use their own clinical judgement and can be flawed if the information received is inaccurate. Many of these systems have 'see GP' as their end-point as in the case of some NHS Direct algorithms.

Case study 1

 Telephone Triage

A call was taken from the mother of a boy aged 8 who had a 2-day history of loose stools and 'tummy' ache. She reported that he was otherwise well, had not been abroad recently and no other family members were ill. She had not seen any blood or mucus in his stools and he had not vomited since the first day. She had encouraged him to drink fluids.

There was no previous medical history of note – all his vaccinations were up to date.

Case study 1 cont'd

Since this was a telephone consultation and visual and physical examination were not possible, the mother's answers had to be relied upon. The boy was responsive, alert, not unduly sleepy and his breathing rate was steady. His skin was warm, not dry and he had no fever; skin colour was normal; mouth was moist; and tongue was not coated.

His abdomen did not appear distended or hard and he was passing wind. Pain was generally lower in his abdomen and not specifically to one side.

He was passing urine normally, his mother had not noticed if this was any darker than usual.

Diagnosis based on the symptoms and signs was viral gastroenteritis. His mother was advised to give clear fluids or flat carbonated drinks for 24 hours, then re-introduce a light bland diet (such as plain toast/boiled rice/plain chapattis). The mother was advised to give him paracetamol suspension 250 mg/5 ml for pain and fever as required, not exceeding the stated dose. The mother was also advised to contact the surgery if he became worse or was not improving after 48 hours.

Had there been any blood in his stools, pain localised to a specific area or undue drowsiness, he would have been seen in surgery.

Differential Diagnoses

Crohns disease, lactose intolerance, cystic fibrosis, chronic non-specific diarrhoea of childhood, winter vomiting disease. These were ruled out by history taking but should symptoms persist the mother had been advised to seek medical attention.

The triage nurse working in a GP surgery has access to the patient's notes, medical history, current medication, allergies and other information but there are disadvantages associated with this type of consultation:

▶ They cannot see the person in front of them.
▶ They are unable to examine the patient; look at a rash; listen to chest sounds in order to formulate a diagnosis.
▶ This can be further compounded if the consultation is a 'third party' call: a worried parent or spouse, a patient whose first language is not english (assuming the triage nurse only speaks english).

▶ A telephone consultation with a patient who has learning difficulties may prove too challenging and if unsure the nurse would advise the patient to attend surgery.

▶ If speech or hearing is impaired another difficult dimension is added.

▶ Explanation of how to take medication, use inhalers or apply dressings might be necessary, in such cases a face-to-face consultation would be more appropriate.

▶ Telephone triage can be abused by patients stocking up on medications, to take on holiday for instance!

▶ Following diagnosis and treatment advice the patient or carer may still need to attend the surgery to collect a prescription or in surgeries with linked pharmacies they will need to collect the medicines.

▶ If there is the slightest shred of doubt or uncertainty concerning a diagnosis or if a demonstration is required it is important to see the patient in the surgery.

▶ 'Near patient' testing may need to be carried out to confirm a diagnosis, or decide if referral into secondary care is required. For example, patients complaining of 'leg pains' could have musculo-skeletal pain, intermittent claudication or a possible deep vein thrombosis and an examination would be necessary with referral if in doubt.

▶ Frequency of micturition could be cystitis, but testing may reveal a urinary tract infection or the onset of diabetes.

Case study 2

A 15-year-old boy with a history of asthma for 8 years telephoned complaining of worsening symptoms. He is on Step 2 of the BTS/SIGN Asthma Treatment Guidelines[9] and has been seen sporadically for asthma. He had been generally healthy and well controlled but during the hay fever season he tends to need his reliever inhaler more frequently. He is a non-smoker.

Symptoms included wheeze, a non-productive cough, worse on exertion and at night. He had recently been camping in the Peak District. His Peak Flow Readings had reduced from 380 to 290. He had doubled up his beclometasone Inhaler, and started two puffs of salbutamol regularly.

Case study 2 cont'd

Over the telephone it was easy to hear that he could speak and string sentences normally, although a slight wheeze could be heard and several times he needed to cough. He explained that he felt warm but did not feel that he had a fever. He had no chest pain or tightness and had used his salbutamol reliever inhaler twice in the past hour with little effect, he had noticed that the inhaler was almost empty and requested a new prescription for this.

Acute exacerbation of asthma was diagnosed in view of his symptoms and reduced peak flow, possibly aggravated by the camping trip. On discussion it was decided to give a short course of oral prednisolone at a dose of 40 mg* daily for 5 days, his weight was 50 kg.[11] He was advised to continue with his increased beclometasone and regular salbutamol. A prescription for all three items was provided.

Differential Diagnoses

Chest infection, pneumonia, foreign body, cystic fibrosis, psychological dyspnoea,[12] acute pneumothorax, tuberculosis.

Telephone consultations improve access and are an acceptable alternative to face-to-face consultations for reviewing patients with symptomatic asthma[13] and managing problems, especially in patients with busy lives like teenagers. They are similar to face-to-face reviews apart from practical procedures like peak flow, height and weight measurements and review of inhaler techniques.

Exercise

Think about the decisions you could make through nurse triage. How could you ensure safety? Find a local policy or guideline relating to triage and write down the key safety points made. Think about your own communication skills. How does your behaviour adapt to the particular situation and the individual patient? How do body language and non-verbal clues influence your approach and your decision-making?

Face-to-Face Triage

The types of patient seen vary immensely. An audit of the author's clinics found that the presenting complaints varied from minor

---

* Dose in children 2–18 yrs 1–2 mg/kg maximum of 40 mg for 3–5 days. Adult dose in acute asthma is 40–50 mg.[10]

self-limiting illnesses like coughs and colds to acute abdominal pain, which resulted in referral to secondary care where a bleeding gastric ulcer was diagnosed.[14] Many patients require simple advice and reassurance, and can be dealt with swiftly such as those with medication queries. Others are more complex, requiring a longer time and/or liaison with other health professionals as in the case of patients returning from abroad with diarrhoea or symptoms suggestive of malaria. Women with gynaecological ailments often present to the nurse particularly in areas with predominantly male GPs.

The NMC states that entries in records should be made contemporaneously.[15] These should provide enough information for another professional to be capable of taking over a patient's care. Entries must be clear, meaningful and unambiguous.[15]

The concept of nurses undertaking a consultation is still relatively new. However, consultation models and skills described in medical literature are relevant to all practitioners. Roger Neighbour[16] describes the consultation as a 'journey not a destination' 'ongoing with the unfolding of symptoms, problems and feelings' some of which may never conclude as there is always another problem, or time, to discuss it. He divides the consultation into five points, which are demonstrated in Table 17.2.

Neighbour's model is useful to apply to triage, despite being developed in 1987. Nurses who see a high proportion of non-English speaking patients without the availability of interpreters often find that it is best to see patients face to face. This can also be the case for patients who have a hearing impairment, those with learning difficulties or mental health problems. Even with the use of a trained interpreter there may be issues relating to translation. The patient's perception of medication and its use may differ from that of the professional's or the interpreter's. Health beliefs may vary considerably, and consideration and sensitivity are necessary to ensure that an understanding is reached.

The benefits of face-to-face consultations include:

▶ direct observation of the patient
▶ ability to check understanding of treatment
▶ ability to pick up non-verbal cues
▶ enabling a more informed diagnosis.

Table 17.2 Neighbour's consultation model 1987[16]

Connecting	Establishing a relationship and building a rapport with the patient, for example greeting, and reflecting on any previous relationship/consultation or review
Summarising	Taking a history, summarising the problem and reflecting it back to the patient to ensure there are no misunderstandings
Handing over	Bringing the consultation to a point where both the patient's and practitioner's agendas are agreed and a management plan is developed
Safety netting	Acknowledging that things may not turn out as planned ensuring that the patient knows what to do if this should happen. For example, the patient with asthma might be advised to take their bronchodilator inhaler regularly and to monitor their peak flows, returning if their peak flow continues to fall or their symptoms worsen
Housekeeping	Tidying away of notes, writing up notes and details, follow-up, and referrals. The practitioner reflects on the consultation. This may involve a debrief with a colleague or merely acknowledging to oneself the effect a particular consultation has had, and, of course, preparing for the next patient

Source: Used with permission from Oxford Radcliffe Medical Press.

The use of prescribing is an essential part of advanced nursing practice. Nurses are able to demonstrate their competence by initiating treatment following diagnosis.

Case study 3

A 5-year-old Indian girl presented with a red, painless 'rash' on face, affecting lips and chin, she was otherwise well. Her mother had applied Vaseline cream.

A past medical history of headlice, chickenpox and constipation was noted, she was up to date with her immunisations.

Initial Observations

The child was thin but not underweight, fully mobile and alert, with fluent speech and not systemically unwell. No other family member had any similar signs.

Case study 3 cont'd

Specific Examination

Skin examined: Several blisters and pustules present to chin and margin of lips with honey coloured, crusted plaques of less than 2 cm with defined margins and minimal or no surrounding redness. No swelling or tenderness of neck lymph glands. A diagnosis of bullous impetigo was made.

Treatment may be topical if localised: fusidic acid (sodium fusidate) can be used, mupirocin ointment three times daily (Prodigy guidance recommends that mupirocin is reserved for second-line therapy). There is some argument as to whether all impetigo lesions should be treated with systemic antibiotics as topical antibiotics are associated with increased antibiotic resistance. Flucloxacillin or erythromycin (if patient is allergic to penicillin) are the oral antibiotics of choice as they are effective against *Staphylococcus aureus* infections.

Gentle debridement of lesions and crusts with a washcloth soaked in warm water and anti-bacterial soap is recommended. Advice about not sharing hand towels or facecloths was given with general advice about handwashing. The children's mother was also reminded that it is contagious and to *keep the children from nursery/school until there is no further crusting*.

Differential Diagnoses

Eczema, ringworm, herpes infection, scabies or impetigo secondary to scabies, impetigo like wound infections. Sometimes the vesicles of impetigo, particularly if dried, can resemble the marks made by cigarette burns, and this can lead to suspicion of deliberate harm and child abuse. If there was the slightest doubt it would be important to refer on to the community paediatricians with responsibility for Child Protection, as soon as possible.

Complications of Bullous Impetigo

▶ scarring
▶ cellulitis, supparative lymphadenitis, furunculosis, abscess, septicaemia
▶ toxic shock syndrome.

Delayed Prescriptions

The changing role of the nurse to that of prescriber can cause additional pressure as she/he may feel pressure to provide a prescription. This can lead to conflict particularly if the patient believes that an antibiotic will make a viral sore throat better, yet evidence shows the contrary.[17,18] These occasions can create less conflict if the nurse issues a 'delayed' or 'post-dated' prescription. Delaying prescription of antibiotics, rather than refusing to prescribe them, is a strategy suggested to address patient expectations and reduce unnecessary use of antibiotics.[19] These prescriptions are either given to the patient, but dated a few days in the future, or the patient is requested to return after three days if the symptoms are not resolved, the medication will then only be dispensed on or after the date on the form.[19] It is recommended that the use of delayed prescriptions should be restricted to those in whom the practitioner feels antibiotics may be indicated in the near future. Concerns around patients representing for the same illness seem to be unfounded. One study found that those given a delayed prescription for antibiotics for a sore throat were 11 per cent less likely to re-attend for a sore throat in the subsequent year than those given an 'immediate' prescription.[20] The rules in relation to nurses giving delayed prescriptions need to be clarified.

Exercise

Many conditions are known to be self-limiting. Think of a condition where you might wish to use a delayed prescription for an antibiotic. Consider the evidence for not prescribing the antibiotic immediately. Does this give you more confidence to use this method in the future?

Conclusion

The nurse–patient encounter is a two-way process with differing agendas which may relate to the receipt of a prescription. The ability to prescribe is a recognition of a nurse's autonomy, diversity of skills and clinical expertise, and the further extension of prescribing rights is giving positive messages about their competence in this area. To enable nurse prescribing to succeed it must be viewed as a proactive measure to assist in the development of a more flexible service for patients.

References

1. Gallagher, M., Huddart, T. and Henderson, B. 'Telephone triage of acute illness by a practice nurse in general practice: Outcomes of care'. *British Journal of General Practice*, 48: 11 (1999) 1141–1145.

2. Lattimer, V., George, S., Thompson, F., Thomas, E., Mullee, M. and Turnbull, J. 'Safety and effectiveness of nurse telephone consultation in out of hours primary care: A randomised controlled trial'. *British Medical Journal*, 317 (1999) 1054–1059.

3. Jones, K., Gilbert, P., Little, J. and Wilkinson, K. 'Nurse triage for house call requests in a Tyneside general practice: Patients' views and effect on doctor workload'. *British Journal of General Practice*, 48 (1999) 1303–1306.

4. Dale, J., Williams, S., Crouch, R. and Patel, A. 'A study of out-of-hours telephone advice from an A&E department'. *British Journal of Nursing*, 6: 3 (1997) 171–174.

5. Dale, J., Crouch, R., Patel, A. and Williams, S. 'Patients telephoning A & E for advice: A comparison of expectation and outcomes'. *Journal of Accident and Emergency Medicine*, 14: 1 (1997) 21–23.

6. Wanless, D. *Securing Our Future Health: Taking a Long-Term View. Final report* (London: HM Treasury, 2002).

7. Richards, D. and Tawfik, J. 'Introducing nurse telephone triage into primary care'. *Nursing Standard*, 15: 10 (2000) 42–45.

8. Farrand, L., Leprohon, J., Kalina, M., Champagne, F., Contandriopoulos, A.P. and Preker, A. 'The role of protocols and professional judgement in emergency medical dispatching'. *European Journal of Emergency Medicine*, 2: 3 (1995) 136–148.

9. British Thoracic Society/Scottish Intercollegiate Guidelines Network (BTS/SIGN). 'Summary of stepwise management of asthma in adults'. *Thorax, International Journal of Respiratory Medicine*, 58 (2003) supp1/24.

10. British Medical Association, Royal Pharmaceutical Society of Great Britain, Royal College of Paediatrics and Child Health, Neonatal and Paediatric Pharmacists Group. *BNF for Children* (London: BMA/RPSGB/RCPCH, 2005).

11. Prodigy. *Prodigy Guidance: Asthma*. 2nd edition (London: The Stationary Office, 2005).

12. Pinnock, H., Bawden, R., Proctor, S., Wolfe, S., Scullion, J., Price, D. and Sheikh, A. 'Accessibility, acceptability, and effectiveness in primary care of routine telephone review of asthma: Pragmatic, randomised controlled trial'. *British Medical Journal*, 326 (2003) 477–479.

13. British Medical Association/Royal Pharmaceutical Society of Great Britain. *British National Formulary* (London: BMA/RPSGB, September 2005).

14. Garratt, S. *Analysis of Triage Clinics* (Unpublished study) Central Derby PCT (2004).

15. NMC. *Guidelines for Records and Record Keeping* (London: NMC, 2005).

16. Neighbour, R. *The Inner Consultation: How to Develop an Effective and Intuitive Consulting Style*. 2nd edition (Oxford: Radcliffe Medical Press, 2004).

17. Prodigy. *Guidance Sore Throat – Acute*. http://www.prodigy.nhs.uk/guidance.asp?gt=Sore%20throat%20-%20acute# Antibiotics, accessed 17/4/05 (2004).

18. Del Mar, C.B. and Glasziou, P. 'Antibiotics for sore throat (Cochrane review).' In: *The Cochrane Library*, Issue 3 (Oxford: Update Software, 1999).

19. Arroll, B. 'Editorial. Delayed Prescriptions'. *British Medical Journal*, 327 (2003) 1361–1362.

20. Little, P., Gould, C., Williamson, I., Warner, G., Gantley, M. and Kinmonth, A.L. 'Re-attendance and complications in a randomised trial of prescribing strategies for sore throat: The medicalising effect of prescribing antibiotics'. *British Medical Journal*, 315 (1997) 350–352.

Chapter 18

Patient group directions, independent and supplementary prescribing

Mike Brownsell

Introduction

This chapter will review current legislative frameworks which support non-medical prescribing, before moving on to differentiate between the uses of patient group directions (PGDs) and non-medical prescribing. Reasons why PGDs may still be preferred over independent and supplementary prescribing will be considered, before concluding with suggestions for the way forward.

Current Legislation

There are five main routes for patients to gain access to medications from a health care professional other than a doctor. These are listed below:

1. **Specific Medicines Act Exemptions**
   These allow certain groups of health care professionals, such as midwives, podiatrists and pharmacists, to sell, supply and/or administer particular medicines directly to patients.[1] By this mechanism, a podiatrist can prescribe, administer, and then charge for a local anaesthetic required when carrying out a minor surgical procedure which may take place in a clinic or the patient's home.

2. **Patient Specific Directions (PSDs)**
   These PSDs consist of written instructions from a doctor, dentist or nurse prescriber for a medicine to be supplied and/or administered to a *named* person. This could be a written request in a

patient's notes or an entry on the patient's drug chart. There is often confusion about when to use a PSD and when to use a PGD. In practice, this is likely to depend on how an individual service is structured. For example, a doctor referring patients to a nurse-led clinic within an acute hospital may write a PSD in a patient's notes for the nurse to administer (and possibly supply) a particular medicine. Alternatively, the same nurse-led clinic may have several PGDs that cover the patient groups likely to be seen in that clinic. Often practical realities such as stock availability and the numbers of trained staff dictate which of these two approaches is taken.

3. **Patient Group Directions (PGDs)**

   These are written instructions that allow some health care professionals to supply and administer a range of medicines directly to patients without the need for a prescription or an instruction from a prescriber in certain circumstances. A PGD is described within various health service circulars across England, Scotland and Northern Ireland[2,3,4] as:

   > a written instruction for the supply and/or administration of named medicines in an identified clinical situation. It applies to groups of patients who may not be individually identified before presentation for treatment.

   It is not a form of prescribing and there is no specific training that health professionals must undertake before supplying medicines in this way.[5] Individual organisations, however, must make sure that health care professionals using PGDs are competent to do so. Importantly, no pharmacist is involved in checking the appropriateness of the medication supplied by the health professional. Pharmacists are an integral part of the committee which formulate the PGDs, but by the very nature of PGD usage, they are not present to check the appropriateness of the medication to a particular patient, as they would be when processing a prescription.

4. **Independent (Non-Medical) Prescribing**

   The prescriber (currently a nurse or a pharmacist) takes responsibility for the clinical assessment of the patient, establishing a diagnosis and deciding the clinical management required. The prescriber is wholly responsible for the prescribing decision. The patient then presents the prescription to a pharmacist who checks and dispenses the medicine against the prescription. This may raise issues when the pharmacist is the one initiating the prescription as the safety checks are once again removed. Medicines law recognises the value of pharmacists in the dispensing process and this is considered the preferred route for patients to obtain their medicines. There were, until very recently, only two types of independent prescribers recognised in law, namely doctors and dentists.

5. **Supplementary Prescribing**

The origins of supplementary prescribing have been discussed in the first two chapters of this book. It is worthwhile re-iterating the definition of supplementary prescribing, defined by the DH as:

> a voluntary prescribing partnership between an independent prescriber and a supplementary prescriber, to implement an agreed patient-specific Clinical Management Plan with the patient's agreement.[6]

In the first instance this prescribing partnership was for nurses and pharmacists. More recently, from 2005, it has been further extended to allow AHPs such as physiotherapists, radiographers, podiatrists[6] and optometrists to prescribe under the same framework.[7]

Exercise

Consider the use of the prescribing behaviours described above. Which of these are being used in your area of work? How do you maintain your competence for the use of any of these methods? Update your professional portfolio with the evidence of this.

Some of the law which governs prescribing is contained within:

- the Medicines Act 1968 (the Primary legislation)[8] and subsequent legislation to Section 58 to include nurses, midwives and health visitors as appropriate practitioners
- the Medicinal Products: Prescription by Nurses and so on Act 1992[9]
- the Health and Social Care Act 2001[10]
- the Misuse of Drugs Regulations 2001.[11]

Subsequent amendments to legislation vary across the United Kingdom and it is important for professionals to know the law that applies to their practice in a particular country.

Within this rapidly changing arena a recent amendment to the Misuse of Drugs Regulations 2001 has been made for inclusion of CDs within the supplementary prescribing framework for nurses and pharmacists from 14 April 2005.[12] This ruling does not as yet apply to allied health professional supplementary prescribers,[6] nor to those practising in countries outside of England. It therefore remains a complex framework, which requires careful navigation by a nurse, pharmacist or AHP wishing to facilitate timely access to medications for patients.

Exercise

Consider the impact that the changes in medicines legislation have had on your area of practice. What are you able to prescribe, through which prescribing route and what is the supporting legislation?

The next part of the chapter will discuss the differences between 'prescribing' and 'supply and administration'. The situation regarding PGDs will be clarified and suggestions will be made as to why nurses and AHPs may sometimes prefer to use PGDs rather than prescribing. Finally the risks and benefits of the use of PGDs and CMPs will also be discussed.

The Current Situation

To 'prescribe' is *to authorise in writing* the supply of a medicine or appliance (usually, but not necessarily, a prescription only medicine (POM) for a *named patient*.

The use of a PGD is *to give, supply or administer a medicine* (qv 'administer' in Section 130 of Medicines Act 1968).[8] A PGD therefore, is an administration tool only, it is *not* prescribing.

Currently doctors are the only unrestricted independent prescribers, although district nurses and health visitors have been independently prescribing for over a decade, and their numbers exceed 28,000.[13] Following training, first-level nurses can now utilise independent prescribing rights from the whole BNF.*

In some areas nurses and AHPs preferred to use PGDs rather than non-medical prescribing as the boundaries for the latter were constantly changing. It imposed restrictions such as: supplementary prescribing involves the formulation of patient specific CMPs that have to be agreed by the independent prescriber, the supplementary prescriber and the patient (or carer). Additionally they need to be supported by protocols and guidelines. Whilst this is good practice it may be time-consuming for busy practitioners, many of whom have found the process too wieldy and supplementary prescribing to date may have been underused in practice.

Pragmatically PGDs may offer more prescribing opportunities for nurses and AHPs in certain roles. Attendance on training programmes for non-medical prescribing requires a huge investment of time. Although money is sometimes available to replace staff, it is difficult to find appropriately trained professionals to cover. A further compounding issue is that around the same time as non-medical prescribing was being discussed, PGDs were formalised in the 1998 'Review of the Prescribing, Supply and Administration of Medicines'. This review recognised the benefits of group protocols and proposed that the law was clarified to ensure that they were being used in a consistent way and that health care professionals working within these protocols were protected legally.

Exercise

Reflect on the administration of medicines in your specialty. Are there any qualified non-medical prescribers or do only doctors prescribe?
How does this affect the patient or client? Do they have to wait and see a doctor if they require a prescription? Is supplementary prescribing used in your area and if so for what conditions?

PGDs were not intended to be a 'first choice' service provision. The Health Service Circular guidance[2,3,4] makes it clear that the majority of clinical care should be provided on an individual,

---

*See Chapter 2 for exceptions to this rule.

patient-specific basis. The supply and administration of medicines under PGDs should be reserved for those limited situations where this offers a significant advantage for the patient without compromising patient safety, such as the administration of analgesia in emergency situations or emergency contraception within an advisory clinic. PGDs are therefore most useful where medicines use can be predicted as the most appropriate way of managing specific episodes of treatment at that time, they are not intended for long-term management of an illness. For nurses working in WICs, or practicing where a medical practitioner is unavailable to act as an independent prescribing partner in a supplementary prescribing partnership, PGDs will remain a useful tool, although non-medical prescribing is a very viable option.

A wide range of professional groups can use PGDs. Since their usage provides effective methods of treating defined groups of patients without access to a doctor, such as road traffic accident victims, they have become a useful tool for paramedics for administering analgesia, oxygen or intravenous fluids. Another patient group who have benefited from the use of PGDs are women requiring post-coital contraception (otherwise known as 'emergency hormonal contraception'). The importance of taking the medication as quickly as possible following unprotected sex and the known reducing efficacy over the following 72-hour period clearly illustrate the potential improvements in service that PGDs can bring.

Professional groups who can use PGDs are:

- midwives
- nurses
- pharmacists
- radiographers
- chiropodists
- ambulance paramedics
- health visitors
- optometrists
- orthoptists
- physiotherapists.

Some professionals are now able to prescribe medicines independently, within the scope of their expertise. Other professional groups can train as supplementary prescribers, these are mentioned in other chapters of this book.

Since information that should be contained in a PGD is complex (unlike the comparatively quick and simple approach adopted for developing a CMP), one would expect this group of professionals to quickly move from PGD use to independent or supplementary prescribing as able. Additionally, when supplying or administering a medicine under a PGD, the patient must fall exactly into the criteria determined by the PGD. If not, the patient must be referred in line with the detailed guidelines. Further information on what should be included can be found in the relevant health service guidance documents.[2,3,4]

In order for the PGD to be legal there are a number of requirements, which must be included.[2] These are shown in Box 18.1.

Box 18.1 Legal requirements of a PGD[2]

- the name of the business to which the direction applies
- the date the direction comes into force and the expiry date
- a description of the medicine(s) to which the direction applies
- class of health professional who may supply or administer the medicine
- signature of a doctor or dentist as appropriate, and a pharmacist
- signature by an appropriate health organisation lead (such as Director of Nursing)
- clinical condition, or situation to which the PGD applies
- description of patients excluded from treatment under the PGD
- details of dosage (including maximum), quantity, form and strength, route and frequency of administration, minimum or maximum period over which the medicine should be administered
- relevant warnings, including potential adverse reactions
- details of any necessary follow-up action
- a statement of the records to be kept for audit purposes.

Source: Health Service Circular 2000/026 © Crown Copyright, 2006.

Some nurses who are now qualified and able to prescribe still report a preference for using PGDs.[14] It is safe to say that even when independent prescribing for individual patients is widespread, there will be times when PGDs will be the best way to meet the patients' needs as they provide the framework for the supply and administration of medicines without the need for an individual prescription and so will remain invaluable in some direct access services and certain emergency situations.[5] Additionally, the burden on service to identify suitably experienced and motivated staff for release to attend a training programme for non-medical prescribing will ensure the use of PGDs remains an attractive option for service managers for some time to come.

As with supplementary prescribing, each professional using a PGD must be a registered member of their profession and act within their appropriate code of professional conduct. They do not need to have successfully completed specific training and be registered before they are allowed to administer medicines. However the National Prescribing Centre points out, organisations using PGDs must designate an appropriate person within the organisation (for example, a clinical supervisor, line manager, general practitioner) to ensure that only fully competent, qualified and trained health care professionals use PGDs and that appropriate training is available.[15] To date, many Trusts have embraced the use of PGDs without fully appreciating the resource implications of the 2-year requirement for regular review, resulting in many health care practitioners inadvertently using a PGD which is past its intended period of effect. Additionally, without an agreed competency framework or training for use, PGDs can lead to inappropriate drug administration to an individual who would not have been prescribed the same drug if other choices were available. A patient may have fitted the criteria, but without robust exclusion criteria, or guaranteed knowledge of such factors as concomitant medication interactions expected of an independent or supplementary prescriber, the potential for patient harm persists.

Exercise

Discuss the risks of using a PGD with your mentor or a colleague. Consider the advantages. Think about how the risks could be minimised. Compare this with the risks of independent prescribing. How can you minimise these risks?

Change within non-medical prescribing has been slow and out of step with how nurses and other health care professionals are modernising health care delivery, and the development and use of PGDs is complex. Nurses attempting to facilitate timely access to medication for patients through the use of PGDs have been known to facilitate administration of a medication to a patient by using another nurse or care assistant to actually administer the drug. PGD administration was never meant to include a third party. Although this can occur legally where the medication is already in the patient's possession, it does not cover medications by injection or medications kept as stock within a secondary care setting. Nurses should not sign for administration of a medication through a PGD and then pass it on to the ward staff to give to a patient.

The most recent consultation commissioned by the DH examined the evidence surrounding prescribing practice. Research has identified that nurses only prescribe within their competency levels.[16] Feedback from patients suggests that nurses support their prescribing with appropriate advice as well as negotiating treatment options with patients to promote concordance.

Practice continues to drive policy, rather than policy guiding practice. Pharmacists have now been granted independent prescribing rights. The key principles of the extension of prescribing responsibilities as laid down by the Department of Health 2002[17] and the National Prescribing Centre[5] include:

- Patient safety is paramount.
- Patients should benefit by enabling faster access to care, including the medicines they need. They should also benefit from having their care actively managed by 'experts' in their condition (for example, specialist nurses and/or pharmacists). This should result in patients receiving more detailed advice on their treatment and a high level of concordance.
- The organisation/service should benefit by making better use of available resources. Maximising the potential of existing skills of a range of health care professionals will increase their contribution to the work of the whole health care team. This means that doctors should have more time to concentrate on those patients who need the level of care that only a doctor can provide.

It is clear that whatever form of prescribing or administration is utilised by health care professionals, providing proper clinical governance processes are in place, the above aims and patient needs can be safely and effectively met. What is required is improved clarity of guidance, and a willingness from the various professional groups to allow health professionals to use the frameworks.

Exercise

Find a PGD either in your work environment or through an appropriate website. Explore the content and reflect on what you have read in this chapter. Write a short account for your professional portfolio analysing whether this has enabled the patient to receive more timely care.

Conclusion

What appears clear is that the use of PGDs is not prescribing. They work best within services where medicines use follows a predictable pattern for an identifiable group of patients for a specific treatment episode. When deciding which approach to take, there remains a need to clarify the purpose of the medicine and whether there is a need for it to be supplied under the terms of a PGD or an individual prescription. PGDs are not appropriate where a health professional needs to take responsibility for managing and clinically responding to an individual patient's condition over the long term, and where a prescribing partnership built on understanding and trust is required to ensure effective monitoring, treatment and patient concordance as with diabetes and hypertension management.

Although clearly a preferred option, the use of independent and/or supplementary prescribing rather than PGD administration is hindered by the lengthy training requirements.

Employees of NHS organisations have indemnity by virtue of vicarious liability whichever method of prescribing is used.[18] Clinical governance and audit surrounding PGD use are local responsibilities, but those same responsibilities relate to independent prescribing by nurses and pharmacists. There is always risk attached to prescribing activity particularly when practitioners are pushing the boundaries of legislation. Recent legislation has legitimised the practice associated with PGD use but care must be taken to ensure that they are updated regularly and used effectively. Health care professionals are advised to take out professional indemnity in addition to relying on vicarious liability cover. The Royal College of Nursing (RCN) does not presently charge extra for cover relating to prescribing but organisations such as the Medical Defence Union (MDU) do. Professionals should ensure that they have adequate cover and that prescribing responsibilities are included in their job descriptions.

References

1. MHRA. *Prescribing, Sale and Supply of Medicines.* www.mhra.gov.uk/inforesources/saleandsupply.htm, accessed 20 July 2005.

2. NHS Executive. *Patient Group Directions* (England Only) HSC 2000/026. www.doh.gov.uk/coinh.htm, accessed 20 July 2005.

3. Scottish Executive. *Guidance: Patient Group Directions.* NHS, HDL (2001), 7. www.scotland.gov.uk, accessed 22 January 2006.

4. DHSSPS. *Guidance: Patient Group Directions.* 7 September 2000. www.dhsspsni.gov.uk, accessed 22 January 2006.

5. NPC *Patient Group Directions: A Practical Guide and Framework of Competencies for All Professionals using Patient Group Directions* (Liverpool: NPC, 2004).

6. DH. *Supplementary Prescribing by Nurses, Pharmacists, Chiropodists/Podiatrists, Physiotherapists and Radiographers within the NHS in England: A Guide for Implementation.* Department of Health website Gateway reference: 4941 (2005). www.dh.gov.uk, accessed 5 May 2005.

7. Potter and Robinson. *Non-Medical Prescribing.* www.npc.co.uk/pdf/Paul%20Robinson%20and%20Claire%20Potter.pdf, accessed 08/07/05.

8. DH. Medicines Act (London: DH, 1968).

9. HMSO. Medicinal Products: Prescriptions by nurses etc. Act 1992 (London: HMSO, 1992).

10. DH. Health and Social Care Act 2001 (London: HMSO, 2001).

11. DH. Misuse of Drugs Regulations (London: HMSO, 2001).

12. DH. The Misuse of Drugs (Amendments) Regulations. Statutory Instrument No. 271 (London: HMSO, 2005).

13. Courtenay, M. and Griffiths, M. *Independent and Supplementary Prescribing: An Essential Guide* (London: Greenwich Medical Media, 2004).

14. DH. *Medicines Matters: A Guide to Current Mechanisms for the Prescribing, Supply and Administration of Medicines* (London: Modernisation Agency, 2005).

15. NPC. MeRec Briefing. No. 23 (Liverpool: NPC, 2004).

16. Latter, S., Maben, J., Myall, M., Courtenay, M., Young, A. and Dunn, N. *An Evaluation of Extended Formulary Independent Nurse Prescribing.* www.nursingandmidwifery.soton.ac.uk/research/grants/latter1.htm, accessed 28 December 2005.

17. NPC. Training Non-Medical Prescribers in Practice: A Guide to Help Doctors Prepare for and Carry out the Role of Designated Medical Practitioner. www.NPC.gov.uk, accessed 9 February 2005.

18. Dimond, B. *Legal Aspects of Nursing.* 3rd edition (Harlow: Pearson Education Ltd, 2002).

Chapter 19

Maintaining competency in prescribing

Millie Smith and Anne Smith

This chapter will discuss the prescriber's responsibility to maintain competency in prescribing, the principles of which equally apply to nurses, AHPs and pharmacists. It will explore issues of maintaining current and competent prescribing knowledge and practice. It will also examine development of the co-requisite skills related to assessment, decision-making and problem solving that are an essential component of the prescribers toolkit.

The key factors that will be examined are:

- regulation
- competence
- organisational responsibility
- personal responsibility for professional development and updating
- transferable skills.

Non-medical prescribing continues to evolve, equipping the practitioner with the skills to develop practice and operate autonomously. Essentially this should enable the patient to receive timely and appropriate care, but conversely if the practitioner fails to update and maintain their proficiency levels, the patient is exposed to risk. The non-medical prescriber has a responsibility both as an individual and as a member of a team to provide safe and effective care.

The policy 'drivers' that influence practice will also be examined as the political climate established by the government has highlighted patient choice[1] and also clearly expressed the role that nurses, pharmacists and AHPs will play in delivering care in different and innovative ways to extend that choice.[2,3] Thus, as new roles are created with new responsibilities it is essential that all health professionals are aware of their accountability and liability in the domain of prescribing.

Professional Regulation

Regulation is an important aspect of any profession. As there are restrictions placed on non-medical prescribers associated with the context of their prescribing and the extent of their role it is imperative that they remain abreast of the changing situation and comply with the regulations that apply to each country within the United Kingdom.

Case study 1

A patient attends a clinic, where they see an allied health professional and they need a prescription for treatment that the AHP is competent to prescribe. The residing doctor and the patient agree to the formulation of a CMP so that the AHP can provide follow-up prescriptions, titration and monitoring of the treatment. The doctor suggests that as he does not have his prescription pad with him that the AHP should prescribe the treatment and they will formulate the plan later that day. The AHP explains that she is unable to do this as this would mean breaching the supplementary prescribing rules but that she would be happy to prescribe at the next visit once the CMP had been formulated and signed. The doctor then obtains a prescription from his office and gives it to the patient. Had he not been able to do this the AHP would still be unable to prescribe prior to the formulation of the CMP as this would be working outside of the supplementary prescribing regulations.

The National Prescribing Centre (NPC) has published a framework to enable practitioners to reflect on practice.[4] It consists of statements that describe competence across a range of categories. The competency areas are divided into sections concerned with:

- the consultation
- prescribing effectively and
- prescribing in context.

Table 19.1 Safe prescribing

Prescribing safely. Is aware of own limitations. Does not compromise patient safety. Knows when to refer or seek guidance from another member of the team or a specialist.	The opportunity to prescribe autonomously from the BNF has implications for non-medical prescribers. While the practitioner may feel qualified to prescribe for a simple presenting problem, the patient may have more complex needs. It is important for the practitioner to undertake a systematic approach to assessment, thereby identifying any concealed symptoms and to understand who will provide support when the prescribing remit is outside the practitioner's role. It is essential to seek appropriate support.

Source: Adapted from the NPC outline framework for nurses.

The NPC outline framework contains statements that describe competence in relation to safe and effective prescribing. This framework is generic and can therefore be adapted to suit the needs of the practitioner relating to the context in which they prescribe. See Table 19.1.

The NMC are currently deliberating over the nurse practitioner role and whether this title should be regulated. There are a number of roles emerging particularly following the publication of the new General Medical Services (nGMS) contract[5] and grave concerns about health professionals adopting more diverse roles with insufficient regulation. Many of these roles include a prescribing remit.[6] Competence is an issue linked to vicarious liability. It is imperative that professionals are conversant with the legal implications of their role and the terms of their employment.[7]

For nurses the NMC Code of Professional Conduct[8] is explicit in detailing the practitioners' responsibility should any harm befall a patient as a result of their actions. Section 9 relates to vicarious liability stating that each practitioner should be aware of the situation with regard to their terms of employment. This can pose problems as the practitioner may lack guidance and support. However, Section 6.3 refers to the obligation on the nurse to seek support and supervision if they lack competence in certain aspects of their role.

The Royal Pharmaceutical Society of Great Britain, RPSGB, states that pharmacists must keep up to date through continuing professional development. In the past this has been obligatory under the Pharmacists Code of Ethics and is expected to become law in 2006.[9] AHPs are also bound by their regulatory frameworks as laid out by the Health Professions Council (HPC). They have 'Standards of Proficiency' for each profession registered with them which can be accessed through their website.[10] The HPC states that 'we were set up to protect your health and wellbeing. To do this, we keep a register of health professionals who meet our standards for their training, professional skills, behaviour and health'.[10]

What is Competence?

At this point it is pertinent to explore the definition of 'competence'. The NMC defines it as 'possessing the skills and abilities required for lawful, safe and effective professional practice without direct supervision'.[8] This is more achievable if a set of benchmark statements are available and this is the rationale for using a generic framework adapted for specialist areas. The benchmark statements articulate the level at which competence or proficiency is achieved. For example, the framework document published by the NPC has an overarching statement within the section relating to 'consultation'.[4] This states that the prescriber 'makes a diagnosis and generates the treatment options for the patient and always follows up treatment' (p. 15). Eleven objectives are then listed which are in effect the benchmark statements.

Exercise

Examine your own practice in relation to this statement. What evidence have you provided of this in your professional portfolio?

The 'consultation' requires the prescriber to demonstrate skills in communication in order to develop a trusting relationship with the client to promote concordance with treatment. See Chapter 21. In relation to consultation a range of competencies are required associated with listening skills, non-verbal communication, observation and use of appropriate language. See Table 19.2.

Table 19.2 The consultation

The consultation	
Communicating with patients Establishes a relationship based on trust and mutual respect. Deals sensitively with patients' emotions and concerns.	The prescriber may reflect that: Having considered the consultation models described in the literature, for example Pendleton, how best to apply these when assessing patients. Often the patient feels uneasy and does not respond accurately about their condition. One of the problems with consultation models such as this is that they are very medically orientated. This may mean that the underlying cause of the problem is not explored as there could be a relationship issue or domestic crisis. Therefore within the consultation it is important to ask open-ended questions and also to wait for the patient's response as it is all too easy to fill the silence rather than allow the patient to answer in their own time.

Source: Adapted from the NPC outline framework for nurses.

Transferable Skills

When debating the issues that determine the competence of the non-medical prescriber, other transferable skills must also be considered. Whilst the focus here may be on the prescribing outcome the practitioner must also possess relevant skills in communication, consultation, assessment and diagnosis. Their decision-making processes will involve a complex combination of judgements based on knowledge within all the domains described within the competency framework.[4] Decisions will encompass actions that are appropriate but will also discard inappropriate actions. The principles of prescribing are not only concerned with generating a prescription. A prescribing decision can take four different routes such as:

- writing a prescription where appropriate
- referral
- recommending over-the-counter medication
- suggesting alternatives associated with reassurance and advice.

The practitioner must be proficient in developing a rapport with the patient and assessing the presenting symptoms in order to make a differential diagnosis. These skills are never static but always developing and it is important for the individual to recognise the merits of reflection and clinical supervision. In this way prescribing will take place within a supportive and critical environment.

Case study 2

A 55-year-old female patient was admitted to hospital for planned surgery. She had suffered from osteoarthritis of her right knee for the past 10 years and mobilising had become extremely difficult. A total knee replacement was to be carried out during this admission. The nurse prescriber seeing the patient notes that she has been taking paracetamol 500 mg, 2 tablets 4 times daily and naproxen 500 mg twice daily. During the admission procedure the nurse was able to prescribe both of these medicines as she was competent in orthopaedic prescribing. The patient stated that she had been depressed as a result of the chronic pain and disability and her GP had prescribed Dothiepin hydrochloride 150 mg daily which she had been taking for the last six months and she requested that the nurse add this to her drug chart as it was important for her to continue this regime. The nurse felt that this was outside of her experience and competence but assured the patient that she would refer this request to one of her medical colleagues before the dose was required that evening. Whilst the nurse was unable to prescribe this medication as it was outside of her competency the patient was able to receive sufficient analgesia for her osteoarthritis and the nurse was able to speak to a medical colleague later that day in order for the patient to receive her other medication. Had the nurse prescribed the dothiepin she would have stepped out of working under her Code of Professional Conduct and her prescribing remit. Conversely, a mental health nurse may be competent to prescribe anti-depressants but may not be competent to prescribe analgesia.

The terms 'competence' and 'competency' are used interchangeably in the literature. However, according to Robotham[11] 'competency' relates to a single activity and 'competence' to a range of competencies. This definition will be used in this chapter.

Race[12] argues that in many instances where competence relates to the acquisition of psychomotor skills the student is only incompetent until educated to perform the skill effectively. He prefers the term 'uncompetence' which he defines as being the state in which a student has not yet become proficient. He finds this term more acceptable and less derogatory when referring to a novice who will attain competence.

The competence levels of practitioners who are making prescribing decisions must be rigorously assessed. There may be some uncertainty about what constitutes competence. Robotham[11] suggests that this term is ambiguous and prefers to use the term 'capability', which has clearer implications. She quotes Ellis[13] with regard to the use of the term 'competence' who states that 'competence is the level beyond which one is incompetent' (p. 252).

Arguably the more aesthetic factors concerned with patient's perceptions are more difficult to quantify and therefore more difficult to assess objectively. This aspect has been included within the framework as some of the benchmark statements examine the practitioner's expertise in teasing out the underlying problems that may be causing symptoms such as anxiety or stress. An example of this is 'does not create a relationship based on prior expectation of a prescription'.

The purpose of the NMC Code of Conduct[8] is to protect the public from incompetent professionals in nursing. It has provided six guiding principles for nurses seeking to extend their roles. These are:

- ensuring that the client's need is uppermost
- keeping up to date
- recognising personal limits of knowledge and skills
- ensuring their expanding role does not encroach on current responsibilities
- acknowledging personal responsibility and accountability
- avoiding inappropriate delegation.

The Health Professions Council will be introducing mandatory CPD requirements from July 2006 and registrants will be required to show evidence of this when requested.[14] Sawbridge[15] suggests three simple rules to ensure practitioner competence

1. They should be suitably trained.
2. They should be aware of and follow established protocols.
3. They should demonstrate continuous professional updating.

Exercise

Consider how frequently you update your portfolio. When did you last make an entry? In what way do you record your updating?

The Department of Health (DH) are cognisant of the fact that this is a relatively new area of work for nurses (even newer for pharmacists and AHPs) and the drivers in primary care are increasing due to the demands of the nGMS contract.[5] Although prescribing responsibility is reportedly to offer patients better choice, the hidden agenda may be more concerned with meeting government targets for patient access. Whilst the DH suggest that patient safety is assured, evidence so far has demonstrated that updating has been patchy and unstructured and has relied on the motivation of the practitioner.[16] Very little attention has been paid to the mechanisms required to maintain competence until recently.[16]

There are a variety of ways in which a practitioner can remain updated, some of which are organised by employers and some which rely on the individual taking personal responsibility. Both parties have an obligation to ensure that the prescriber is operating safely and effectively. The employer bears vicarious liability and the practitioner is accountable within their Code of Conduct.[8] The DH document[2] reinforces the employer's responsibility to provide access to relevant updating.

Personal Responsibility

Continuing professional development is an individual responsibility and as such health professionals are familiar with ways of updating knowledge. Many organisations provide 'in service' courses and study days as a means of updating prescribing. Opportunities may be given to attend local or national conferences that offer expert speakers and provide the opportunity to hear the very latest in developments and emerging ideas. Study days and conferences are probably the best known mechanisms for gaining knowledge and are generally considered to be methods of continuing education. Conferences can be expensive and should be carefully chosen to gain maximum value. Prescribers need to examine the extent of their own knowledge in relation to the programme for the event, looking at the topics and the expertise of speakers before making a decision to attend.

Informal Opportunities for Personal Updating

There are, however, many more opportunities to learn that do not involve formal arenas, are just as valuable and more readily available, and these can be major contributors to continuing professional development.

Exercise

> Reflect on an informal approach that you have adopted to ensure that you have updated your knowledge in prescribing practice. What new knowledge have you gained and how have you used it in practice?

Hancox[17] differentiates between continuing education and continuing professional development regarding the former as a limited means of learning. He explains the difference between these two suggesting that significant learning occurs from day-to-day practice and that this can either be marginalised in the concept of continuing education or developed in the concept of continuing professional development. Continuing education infers that learning takes place through formal study. Continuing professional development takes a wider approach to learning from everyday situations. This can be achieved through using reflection and clinical supervision to find solutions to problems and follow up on questions and comments that are raised by colleagues. It is important to view learning in its widest sense.

Exercise

> Reflect on an informal approach that you have adopted to ensure that you updated your knowledge in prescribing practice. What new knowledge have you gained and how have you used it in your workplace?

Reflective Practice

Health professionals are encouraged to use reflection. Schon[18] refers to reflection in action, reflecting on activities as they occur, and reflection on action which is a deliberate act that takes place after the event. Reflection is a valuable way of learning as it demands personal thoughts and analysis, involving recognition of learning by identifying good practice. It also identifies practice where changes may be needed to improve a situation. Important considerations when prescribing are the ability to analyse and evaluate reasoning that led to prescribing decisions. Thompson[19] in opening remarks in her book on critical reasoning comments that it is not possible to evaluate someone's reasoning if either the words or the reasons offered are not understood. Reflection may help health professionals to analyse their actions and interpret them to others. A reflective diary that documents learning experiences, some of which occur in prescribing may be a useful method of recording this and evaluating learning.

Exercise

Think about the last time that you wrote a reflective account. Did it help you analyse the issues? Was it difficult to articulate your feelings?

The concept of continually reflecting on practise is captured in the NPC framework[4] within the section on 'Improving prescribing practice' (p. 16) encouraging practitioners to adopt an open approach to learning both formally and oppurtunistically.

Professional practice provides a wealth of opportunities to learn, this is often serendipity learning where a new experience or another approach to work brings with it new learning. In the course of normal activity people work with other practitioners and have the opportunity to learn from them. Learning from peers is common practice. Each professional brings different experiences, knowledge, skills, views and values to their work and through working together, observing each other and discussing patient/client care, continuing professional development occurs without conscious effort. This informal but valuable learning should be realised and acknowledged as a way of learning.

Exercise

Discuss with a colleague how an experience in practice has provided a learning opportunity. Have you encountered a significant incident that has triggered a change in practice?

Web-based Learning and Communication

The World Wide Web offers opportunities for practitioners to have direct access to the latest policy guidance, prescribing changes and for peer support. The technology can update practitioners with new information concerning their prescribing rights and opportunities as they are initiated. The virtual environment extends the opportunities for peer support and discussion. There are major advantages to this type of communication. Time constraints associated with meeting face to face for information dissemination or group-based activity is reduced as are travelling costs and staff replacement costs. Generally the idea is that practitioners can access the Internet from their work base causing minimal disruption to their working day and yet enabling them to communicate with other professionals on a global basis if so desired.

Websites are available to provide information and support such as PRODIGY[20] and NPC.[4] The provision of a dedicated website can enable practitioners to communicate across organisational boundaries regarding their experiences and to learn of innovations and barriers accordingly.[21]

Organisational Responsibilities

The health service has a rich supply of information that can be utilised for professional development. An important part of keeping up to date is to have a good knowledge of the sources of information available. Some of these will be national, for example the DH, the NPC and Prescribing Analysis and CosT (PACT)[22] data. There is also local information developed within organisations, for example many NHS Trusts publish prescribing formularies and updating bulletins for staff. Textbooks and journals add to the knowledge base as does comment and opinion.

Appraising the Evidence

The acquisition of new information should always be accompanied by a critical review to establish the validity of the information presented. Evidence-based practice relies on sound evidence and the ability of readers to determine the strength of evidence.[23] Rapid and constant changes make current information essential in any aspect of health care. Reading and searching databases are a means by which evidence-based knowledge is established and maintained. This can be a daunting task but may be made easier by sharing the responsibility between colleagues with each person taking responsibility for reviewing specific sources of information and sharing it with others. This can be achieved through working groups, journal clubs, as part of team meetings or through local publications.

Networking

Developing a network of prescribers can have wide value across the prescribing community. In effect this can be real or virtual. A network has been described as a system that links together people and departments enabling them to share information and resources.[24] As far as continuing professional development is concerned a who's who of prescribing would provide a baseline from which to develop other initiatives. The potential resources within organisations are increasing as the professions who are involved in prescribing expand. Each group of professionals brings its own body of knowledge with different perspectives and approaches to treatment in health care.

The implications of the expansion of the virtual world are being experienced in all areas of peoples' lives and this should be harnessed and utilised to best advantage. Its major advantage is that of linking professionals from a variety of geographical locations to share their experiences, creating a forum for discussion and critical appraisal.[21] There are still many aspects of non-medical prescribing that remain ambiguous. Policy and practice issues continue to be considered and scrutinised. Hence the potential of this support mechanism.

Exercise

Access a prescribing website. Use the communication facility to contact a prescriber from another part of the country.

Networks are particularly suitable for problem solving and questioning as it is usually possible to find someone who has the expertise required, fairly quickly. Thus, not only is the problem solved, it is accompanied by learning. The informality that can develop through networking with people is very much a part of meeting prescribing competencies that relate to working with other members of the prescribing team.[7] Networks can be loose in that they are based on a group of people who have prescribing knowledge and who can be easily contacted. They can also have a more structured style where there is a purpose to meetings with terms of reference that provide a forum for professionals to meet on a regular basis for discussion and updating of prescribing knowledge.

The value of networks is that a whole range of expertise is available on an informal basis. Thus the cost to the organisation is negligible. The cost of updating will always need to be considered and this method of continuing professional development can be attractive to employers as it is not costly in terms of course fees, travelling expenses and staff time away from their workplace.

Continuing professional development, though an individual responsibility, is a partnership between the individual and the organisation for which they work. The individual has a professional responsibility to be up to date with current knowledge and skills. The organisation bears the responsibility for providing the means of acquiring current knowledge as a part of the commitment to provision of health services and employment of staff.

A further suggestion by Hancox[17] relating to continuing education for pharmacists is that those who rely solely on attending courses may be unaware of the gaps that exist in their knowledge. This is an interesting comment in that it infers that simply being offered new information is not sufficient in itself to be considered as professional updating. Courses and conferences have specific topics and that is fine if it is what the person needs. It may, however, be useful to reflect on how often you have come away from a study day or conference feeling disappointed that you have not gained more from it.

Exercise

Reflect on the last study day that you attended. Did you set yourself outcomes prior to attending? List the learning outcomes that you achieved. Record this in your Personal Professional Portfolio.

Conclusion

Health service organisations are increasingly juggling competing priorities. There are constant demands from the provision of new technology, new treatments, new findings in evidence-based care that must be implemented and health policy that directs new ways of working and sets NHS Trusts targets that must meet.[25] All of this and limited resources make it essential to be creative in ways that can be employed to update prescribing knowledge.

Non-medical prescribers are invariably charting new territory and do not have role models to aspire to. They must consider their practice in relation to the principles identified within the clinical governance framework.

The PACT[20] data offers employers the opportunity to examine prescribing patterns and prescribing behaviour. This also indicates the cost-effectiveness of prescriptions raised. The evaluation published in June 2005 indicated that nurses are effective in their role.[26]

There has already been a paradigm shift in custom and practice in relation to the areas of governance. This is particularly noticeable in respect to shared learning where innovative schemes have been created to enable multi-professional 'protected learning time' to be organised.

The major implication of the prescribing remit is that role autonomy is increased and practitioners are able to complete episodes of care by generating a prescription if required. However, as the boundaries are continuously being challenged individuals should always be aware that they are professionally accountable for their actions. It is imperative that they consider their role expansion in relation to effectiveness of patient outcomes and also in consideration of their contractual arrangements.

References

1. Department of Health. *Building on the Best: Choice, Responsiveness and Equity in the NHS* (London: HMSO, 2003).

2. Department of Health. *Liberating the Talents: Helping Primary Care Trusts and Nurses to Deliver the NHS Plan* (London: HMSO, 2002).

3. Department of Health. *Liberating the Public Health Talents* (London: HMSO, 2003).

4. National Prescribing Centre. *Nurse Prescribing Competencies*. www.npc. nhs.uk (Liverpool: NPC, 2004).

5. NHS Confederation, British Medical Association. *The New GMS Contract: Investing in General Practice* (London: The NHS Confederation, 2003).

6. Department of Health. *Supplementary Prescribing by Nurses, Pharmacists, Chiropodists/Podiatrists, Physiotherapists and Radiographers within the NHS in England* (London: DH, 2005).

7. Caulfield, H. 'Responsibility, accountability and liability in nurse prescribing'. *Prescribing Nurse* (Summer 2004).

8. Nursing and Midwifery Council. *The NMC Code of Professional Conduct: Standards for Conduct, Performance and Ethics* (NMC: London, 2004).

9. Royal Pharmaceutical Society of Great Britain. Continuing professional development. www.rpsgb.org.uk/members/cpd/index.html, accessed 8 January 2006.

10. Health Professions Council. Standards of proficiency. www.hpc-org.uk, accessed 8 January 2006.

11. Robotham, A. 'Assessment of competence to practice'. In: Sines, D., Appleby, F. and Raymond, B. (eds) *Community Health Care Nursing*. 2nd edition (Oxford: Blackwell Science, 2001).

12. Race, P. *Never Mind the Teaching Feel the Learning* (Birmingham: SEDA Publications, 2001).

13. Ellis, R. (ed.) *Professional Competence and Quality Assurance in the Caring Professions* (London: Chapman Hall), cited in Robotham, A. 'Assessment of competence to practice'. In: Sines, D., Appleby, F. and Raymond, B. (eds) *Community Health Care Nursing*, 2nd edition (Oxford: Blackwell Science, 2001).

14. HPC. CPD: key decisions (August 2005). www.hpc-org.uk, accessed 8 January 2006.

15. Sawbridge, Y. 'We must be clear about responsibility'. *Independent Nurse*, www.independentnurse.co.uk, accessed 24 January 2005.

16. Brookes, D. 'Selecting and developing extended nurse prescribers'. *Nurse Prescribing*, 2: 5 (2004) 212–216.

17. Hancox, D. 'Making the move from continuing education to continuing professional development'. *The Pharmaceutical Journal*, 268: 7180 (2002) 26–27.

18. Schon, D. *The Reflective Practitioner* (London: Maurice Temple Smith Ltd, 1991).

19. Thompson, A. *Critical Reasoning: A Practical Introduction* (London: Routledge, 1996).

20. Prodigy. (Practical support for clinical guidance) www.prodigy.nhs.uk/nurse

21. Smith, A. 'The use of the internet to support the education of nurse prescribers'. *Nurse Prescribing*, 2: 2 (2004) 127–130.

22. Prescription Pricing Authority. *Prescribing Analysis and CosT Standard Report.* www.ppa.nhs.uk (2004).

23. Gom, R., Needham, G., Bullman, A., *Evaluating Research in Health and Social Care* (London: Sage in association with the Open University, 2000).

24. Daft, R. *Management.* 4th edition (Fort Worth: Dryden Press, 1998).

25. Department of Health. *Prescribing: A Supplement to the CNO Bulletin* (January 2004).

26. Latter, S., Maben, J., Myall, M., Courtenay, M., Young, A. and Dunn, N. *An Evaluation of Extended Formulary Independent Nurse Prescribing* (DH and University of Southampton, 2005).

Useful websites

Nurse Prescriber	www.nurse-prescriber.co.uk
Department of Health	www.dh.gov.uk
PRODIGY	www.prodigy.nhs.uk/nurse
NPC starter CD-ROM available from	www.npc.nhs.uk
Pharmacists	www.rpsgb.org.uk
Allied Health Professionals	www.hpc-org.uk
NHS Education for Scotland	www.nes.scot.uk/nursing/prescribing/

Chapter 20

Patient reflection on nurse prescribing

Anon

As a patient at an all-male doctor's surgery I have found the help and advice from the female nurse practitioner extremely valuable, and have used this service on a number of occasions where, if this was not available, it would have been difficult for me to discuss my medical condition with the male doctors.

This I feel is partly because I am of Asian origin and so are my male doctors. Both of my doctors are Muslim and I am a Sikh and there are some cultural differences and some issues are difficult to speak to them about. This means that sometimes for sensitive issues like those around child bearing and contraception and female problems, we Asian ladies have to register with different surgeries with a female doctor in those cases, this means that a continuous medical service is not provided.

Over the past two years, I have seen my nurse practitioner on a number of occasions, beginning with issues when my husband and I were trying to conceive. I had moved to live here with my husband's family – as is the traditional Indian way – and, aside from my mother-in-law, had no female friends to chat with about babies and my health. I was given a nurse practitioner appointment because it was at a convenient time for me – I worked full time then and none of the doctor's appointments were available. The reception staff gave me a choice of seeing a female nurse practitioner and I was glad to have this opportunity. We had a nice chat about my anxieties and discussed sex, conception, and my general health in an open, honest way, I was advised of the 'ideal' fertile times to have sex with my husband and the nurse practitioner suggested that I should consider having some folic acid tablets – explaining why they were beneficial in pre-conception and early pregnancy. She ascertained that I actually paid for prescriptions then as I was employed, and suggested it might be better to buy them over the counter at the pharmacy as they were not expensive. Once I suspected that I was pregnant, I attended, along with my husband, to see her again to have this confirmed, and I was able to have the test taken there and then, the date our baby would be due was worked out, and my first midwife appointment was arranged.

In the early stages of my pregnancy I was bleeding for several weeks and a number of investigations needed to be carried out to determine why. A number of times I had seen the emergency doctors at the on-call surgery (not my own doctors). Each time I went there because the bleeding had got much worse they would tell me that I was having a miscarriage and would generally give me the brush off. In the end my own GP suggested that I should have a swab taken, and that I would probably feel better if it was taken by my nurse practitioner. He was right of course! She reassured me that everything would be OK and that the procedure would not be harmful, and that sometimes bleeding in early pregnancy does occur to a lot of women, she also suggested that the bleeding might be due to an infection, and when the results from the swab were back this was confirmed.

It was brilliant to get a prescription there and then when I returned for the results and I didn't have to wait for the doctor to come and write it. She took time to explain how to use the treatment that she had prescribed and she wanted to be sure that I would use it correctly so that it would benefit me. I have seasonal asthma. While I was pregnant it was well controlled, but it seemed to be getting worse again at the end of last year.

I went to see the nurse practitioner and we had a long chat about how I managed with my asthma and what effect it had on my life, luckily most of the time I'm OK but occasionally it seems to flare up, sometimes if I'm stressed. She did a full review of my asthma, examined my chest and took some tests to see if it was worse, which it was. She was then able to issue me with some steroid tablets and repeat inhalers, she explained that she was formulating a Management Plan which would stay in my notes and allow her to review my medication, add to it if necessary, and treat me according to the asthma step-wise treatment – this again saved me the time of seeing the doctor and I was able to obtain my prescription.

I've most recently been to see her with regard to family planning; our son is now nine months old. We discussed all of the options available and then decided on two different routes which I felt were best for me. I was given all of the advice I needed to make a decision, and chose the contraceptive pill since I've no plans for a second child yet! This was so much easier to discuss with another woman than a man! (I probably would not have even thought about talking about it with my doctors.) I was then given my nurse prescription there and then and I have been able to go back and discuss any worries about starting the pill with her.

I have found the availability of the nurse practitioner who can prescribe to be a brilliant addition to my doctors' surgery. The appointment times are convenient for myself and other family members, and we are able to be assured of seeing her on the same day if necessary and avoiding a long wait to be seen.

When it comes down to patient choice I would now much prefer to see my nurse practitioner than the GP as she can provide a one-stop medical service: carrying out procedures and tests, and writing up a prescription. This helps both us patients and the doctors. First, for the patient it means there is no waiting about for the prescription, and secondly for the doctor they can spend more time with patients who need it and it relieves their pressures.

It's great being able to see the nurse practitioner and I feel at ease discussing my worries with her – it's like speaking to a good friend. More importantly she has taken time to listen, this is something that sometimes the GPs don't have the time to do owing to the pressures on them and the number of patients that they see. This is an invaluable service that my family and I will continue to use for the foreseeable future. Thank You.

Chapter 21

Consultation skills

Ruth Lonsdale

Introduction

This chapter will consider consultation skills and how they can be managed. The first question to be answered is 'how long is a consultation meant to last'? The length of time that is appropriate will depend on how long it takes to obtain the history, make a differential diagnosis, examination to confirm or refute this and provide a safety net. Clinicians in different settings will take varying amounts of time to achieve the above stages. This is due to having or not having full access to medical records and the general health of the patient. Although there are exceptions, most patients attending GP surgeries are in better health than those patients who are housebound. Consultations therefore vary between 7 minutes and an hour and a half.

Communication in Consultation

The common ground between all clinicians is the need for good communication skills. These enhance the consultation or can create barriers if communication is poor. Various definitions of communication exist:

- Communication is the transmission of a message via speaking, writing or by non-verbal means.[1]
- Messages are conveyed via language, the spoken word, paralinguistic features, which relate to the pace, emphasis, intonation, pitch, rhythm and tone of the voice and body language which relates to facial expression, gaze, posture, body space, touch and dress.[2]

In communication more emphasis is placed on non-verbal cues rather than verbal communication. According to Mehrabian the meaning of messages are conveyed in the following proportions:[3]

- verbal   7 per cent
- non-verbal   38 per cent
- facial expression   55 per cent.

One form of communication is referred to as therapeutic communication.[4] Therapeutic communication is purposeful, providing the patient with a safe place to explore the meaning of the illness.[5] This is important in health care because it supports, educates and empowers patients to cope with health-related issues. Information and emotional support are given so that maximum well-being is achieved.[5] The effect of therapeutic communication with patients is 'a participatory process, listening not only for facts but also underlying meanings of communication with attached values, attributes and feelings'.[6] Examples of unusual speech patterns may be noted as thick accents, rapid or slow speech, monotone voice, high-pitched laughter or rambling.[4] Silence, on the other hand, has been described as a powerful listening response whereas a silent pause is merely a brief disconnection in the dialogue followed by verbal comment.[4] Having considered the differences in types of communication including language issues, the theoretical models of consultation skills will now be discussed.

Models of Consultation

There are a number of models such as the Calgary–Cambridge model[7] that can be used to formulate consultations. This model has five stages namely:

1. Initiating the session
2. Gathering information
3. Building the relationship
4. Explanation and planning and
5. Closing the session.

It is similar to Roger Neighbour's model that also has a five-point check.[8] The five points are as follows:

1. *Connecting*	Establishing a rapport with the patient
2. *Summarising*	Why has the patient come, consider concerns, expectations and then summarise it back to the patient
3. *Handing over Agendas (clinician and patient – both will have one)*	Need to negotiate it and influence it where needed
4. *Safety net*	Consider all the problems that is, 'what happens if . . . '
5. *Housekeeping*	Finished one consultation – am I ready for the next one?

Source: Used with permission from Oxford Radcliffe Press.

In general practice the above models can be used effectively. Clinics/sessions run to time with the ten-minute appointment slot. Establishing a rapport can be rapid. As a clinician, one can and does ask the question 'why have you come today?' In asking this one wishes to establish what parameters in the patient's life have changed so that he/she has come today, not tomorrow and not next week. Sometimes there are underlying reasons and one needs to establish the facts. The agenda, often called the 'hidden agenda', will not be picked up within the consultation unless a rapport has been satisfactorily established and communication skills are adequate. This will involve asking both open and closed questions as well as being conscious of body language. The agenda could be to get the patient to focus on what self-help is available for their current condition. This could be to stop smoking, lose weight or take up exercise. The patient's agenda may be to ignore the health promotion advice and just get some medication so life can continue without disruption. The treatment plan needs to be negotiated with the clinician influencing what is done but allowing the patient to make the ultimate decision. The 'what if . . . ' needs to be considered. In terms of the asthmatic patient the 'what if' will be to consider what to do if symptoms become worse and the medication is not successful. Finishing the consultation is an art in itself. Time is limited. Printing off a prescription (if appropriate) helps to end the consultation but so to does the change in tone of voice and body language.

Table 21.1 The model of therapeutic communication/intervention[9]

Authoritative category	Facilitative category
Prescriptive – giving advice or instructions being critical or directive	*Cathartic* – seeking to release emotion in the form of weeping, laughter, trembling or anger
Informative – imparting new knowledge, instructing or interpreting	*Catalytic* – encouraging the patient to discover and explore his own latent thoughts and feelings
Confronting – challenging a restrictive attitude or behaviour, giving direct feedback within a caring context	*Supporting* – offering comfort and approval, affirming the patient's intrinsic value.

Source: Reproduced with permission from Radcliffe Medical Press.

The model of therapeutic communication/intervention,[9] which has six stages, is described in Table 21.1. The various stages within the categories are not fixed in the order they should appear within the consultation but rather their boundaries remain permeable.[9] This is so the flow through each stage can occur whenever necessary during the consultation enhancing the process.

This model is useful when working with individual patients or with patients and their families. In a setting such as a WIC, patients present with minor illnesses and injuries. Having looked at the theoretical models that can be used, the chapter will now consider the medical aspects of the consultation and any frameworks that can help in the process of finding out the evidence on which decisions can be based.

Case study 1

Brian has sustained an injury to his right foot while playing football. As he is normally fit, well and mobile, the scenario can be applied to minor injuries units, WICs and general practice surgeries. In conducting the consultation, a standard framework commonly known as the 'medical model' will be used interjected with explanations as to how Heron's model of therapeutic communication/intervention might work.[9] It is important to record accurately the mechanism of injury and to ensure a full history is obtained using a symptom sorter framework. Two such frameworks or pneumonics are PQRST[10] and SOCRATES.[11] These can be seen in Tables 21.2 and 21.3, respectively.

Case study 1 cont'd

Table 21.2 Explaining PQRST

P	Provocative or palliative	First occurrence – what were you doing at the time? What trigger aggravates it? What relieves the problem?
Q	Quality or quantity	How would you describe the symptom (feels/looks/sounds)? How often are you getting it? (what does it prevent you from doing?)
R	Region or radiation	Region – where does the symptom occur? Radiation – in case of pain, does it spread anywhere?
S	Severity scale	Severity – how bad is the symptom at its worst? Is the symptom getting better, worse or staying the same?
T	Timing	Onset – on what date did the symptom first occur and what time? How did it start – sudden or gradual? Frequency – how often hourly? daily? weekly? monthly? At what time – day or night? Does it wake you up? Does it occur before, during or after meals? Is there a seasonal variation? Duration – how long does it last?

Table 21.3 Showing the SOCRATES framework

S	Site
O	Onset
C	Character
R	Radiating
A	Alleviating/associated systems
T	Timing
E	Exacerbating/relieving factors
S	Severity

In calling Brian into the consultation room, it is important to notice his general appearance. Although it may not be known why he is come, his stance and walking will also be noted. On this occasion, he has a pained expression on his face and he is limping on his right foot. The SOCRATES framework will be used during the history section in order to establish the nature of the pain and injury.

Case study 1 cont'd

PC – Presenting complaint
Injury to right foot

HPC – History of presenting complaint (Descriptive)
Brian states that whilst playing football his opponent goes for the ball at the same time as himself. This results in a collision when he falls to the floor having hurt his ankle *(onset)*. The mechanism of injury is an inversion injury to the right foot. The *site* has been stated as the ankle but is this he really means? On asking him to point to the pain he points to the side and top of his foot. Although the *timing* occurred during a football match it was actually yesterday that it happened and he had walked on it immediately afterwards and all day today. *Character* of the pain is an ache while sitting, a bit worse on walking, unable to run because of the pain and has not taken any analgesia. There is no spread *(radiating)* of the pain. *Associated symptoms* are that his foot has become more swollen and bruised. Nothing has been tried to relieve the pain. *Exacerbating symptoms* are when he tries to run he gets more pain. Nothing else makes it worse. When asking about severity he says that he has no pain when sitting and only some when walking; however, he is limping. To gauge the *severity* you ask him if 10 is the worst pain he has ever had and 0 is no pain at all where does his pain fit now? He says it is 4. During this process analgesia should be provided if required. This is very useful as Crowther states that physical discomfort, in this instance pain, halts communication and makes listening more difficult.[12]

The rest of the medical model includes the following:

▶ Past medical history and past surgical history
▶ Medication history (including over the counter preparations)
▶ Allergies
▶ Systemic enquiry – questions pertaining to each of the body systems e.g. cardio-vascular system
▶ Social history
▶ Family medical history
▶ Examination
▶ Differential diagnoses
▶ Investigations

Confirmed Diagnosis
Ankle sprain (Informative)

Case study 1 cont'd

Treatment (Confrontation and supporting)

On advising that he rest he laughs (*Cathartic*). He expresses his need to keep fit despite the injury, and as long as nothing is broken he is ok (*Catalytic*). We acknowledge that he wants to continue to work, so rest at lunchtimes and in the evenings is agreed. Ice applied for 20 minutes 4 times daily may help, provided it is wrapped up in a towel first. He may wish to use a bandage for additional support. A patient suffering from asthma may not be able to take ibuprofen as some asthmatics react to non-steroidal anti-inflammatory drugs (NSAIDs) which can exacerbate the condition. An alternative analgesic is paracetamol 500 mg 1–2 tablets 4 times daily *(Prescriptive)*. Safety netting should be provided which means stating that if symptoms are unresolved despite these measures he should return for a review. Depending on where this consultation has happened it may be possible to book an appointment for a review as a normal part of the course.

Case study 2

An 89-year-old lady who is known to the community matron (CM) requests a visit due to increasing breathlessness and feeling unwell. In considering this situation the Calgary–Cambridge model[7] will be used in conjunction with the medical model, PQRST will be used to sort the symptoms.

The patient is having trouble with her breathing and has been admitted to hospital three times this year. In keeping with the above model the CM will need to do the following:

- ▶ initiate the session
- ▶ build the relationship
- ▶ gather information
- ▶ explanation and planning
- ▶ close the session.

Initiating the Session

With every consultation, introductions should always be made. The public have a right to know who is treating them and it is courtesy. The clinician needs to know who the patient is so that the correct patient is identified. When the patient and health professional know each other, the session is initiated through the exchange of greetings.

Case study 2 cont'd

Building the Relationship

Open and closed questions are asked, both medical and social, allowing the patient to express her views whilst obtaining the necessary clinical information and building up a rapport.

Gathering Information

PC
Difficulty in breathing

HPC
- **(P)** Impact on mobility, cough, sputum, pain, alleviating and exacerbating factors
- **(Q)** How often breathless? coughing? worse in morning or at night? amount of sputum? colour?
- **(R)** Pain or discomfort spreading anywhere else?
- **(S)** How does it compare to other exacerbations or use numerical scale?
- **(T)** When it began?

Explanation and Planning

During this phase the clinical examination would be conducted. This will enable the correct amount of information to be given allowing the patient time to accurately recall and understand what has been said and done. This aids a shared understanding of the problem and includes the CM looking at it from the patient's perspective. Shared decision-making is then facilitated.

Closing the Session

The session would then close having reached a satisfactory agreement. Safety netting would then be put in place. It is envisaged that the patient would then be followed up by the CM.

Conclusion

In reviewing the consultation skills chapter, it has not been possible to look at each system and say how to assess it, rather this is a taster of how consultations can be conducted. The author would refer readers to clinical skill text books in order for the full examination skills to be learnt. Frameworks for sifting and sorting symptoms are useful in all consultations although the author appreciates that these two scenarios may not be appropriate for all clinicians. In using frameworks the history taking skills of the clinician will be improved/enhanced. The underlying principles of these and of the models are transferable to all clinical situations.

References

1. Oxford University Press. Oxford Compact English Dictionary (Oxford: OUP, 1996).

2. Ellis, R.B., Gates, R.J. and Kenworthy, N. *Interpersonal Communication in Nursing: Theory and Practice.* 4th edition (Toronto: Churchill Livingstone, 1995).

3. Mehrabian, A. *Silent Messages* (California: Belmont, 1971).

4. Arnold, E. and Underman Boggs, K. *Interpersonal Relationships: Professional Communication Skills for Nurses* (St Louis: Saunders, 1999).

5. Pearson, A., Borbasi, S. and Walsh, K. Practicing nursing therapeutically through acting as a skilled companion on the illness journey. *Advanced Practice Nursing Quarterly*, 3:1 (1997) 46–52.

6. Bush, K. Do you really listen to patients? *Registered Nursing*, 64:3 (2001) 35–37.

7. Kurtz, S. and Silverman, J. The Calgary-Cambridge Approach to Communication Skills Teaching. www.gp-training.net/training/consultation/consulta.htm, accessed on 29 April 2005 (1996).

8. Neighbour, R. *The Inner Consultation: How to Develop an Effective and Intuitive Consulting Style.* 2nd edition (Oxford: Radcliffe Publishing, 2005).

9. Heron, J. Helping the client. *A Creative Practical Guide* (London: Sage Publications, 1997).

10. John Hopkins University. The Art of History Taking. http://www.bme.jhu.edu/~rcheong/Year2/clinicalskills/History%20and%20 Physical%20Exam.doc, accessed 27 February 2006.

11. Browse. Surgery – general history taking principles. SOCRATES. www.geocites.com/idevanat/historytakingprinciples, accessed 26 February 2006.

12. Crowther, D. Metacommunications: A missed opportunity. *Journal of Psychosocial Nursing & Mental Health Services*, 29:4 (1991) 13–16.

Significant steps have been taken in recent years in legislating for the prescribing rights of health care professions other than doctors and dentists. This has not been an easy passage, demonstrated by the protracted timescale involved. Who knows what the future will hold? The NHS is changing beyond recognition, and the extension of prescribing rights for professionals other than nurses has taken a decade to introduce. The latest consultation document resulted in the whole formulary becoming available to nurses and pharmacists but this has been viewed with some scepticism and concern by medical colleagues. The number of practitioners qualified to prescribe is monitored by the Prescribing Support Unit (www.ic.nhs.uk). They indicate that the training targets established at national level are short of those predicted or expected, although prescribing courses throughout the United Kingdom are becoming much more popular since the expansions discussed throughout this book. Much of the confusion around what nurses can prescribe has been eradicated with the latest expansion of the formulary, although it will be even more critical that nurses only prescribe within their level of competence. There is anecdotal evidence that some employing organisations may impose their own restrictions on independent prescribing by nurses. Supplementary prescribing partnerships are likely to continue for some time while nurses and doctors negotiate this momentous change in prescribing practice. Prescribing by other groups of non-medical prescribers will also need to be considered within an established governance framework that supports accurate reporting and continuous updating to maintain knowledge and competence levels. The professional bodies will be best placed to monitor prescribing behaviour linked to professional accountability.

This text has given the reader an impression of the development of prescribing for professions other than doctors and dentists. The dilemmas encountered have been described. Prescribing rights are constantly expanding. The nurses who have been the pioneers in practice have demonstrated that it is effective in increasing patient satisfaction and cost-effective in respect of the NHS budget.[1] It is also effective in developing new ways of working necessary since the introduction of the nGMS contract[2] and the new rules relating to junior doctors working hours.

The government targets associated with out of hours[3] service provision and the management of long-term conditions[4] are clearly linked to the prescribing agenda. Patient access to services is also a key driver[5] and many of the practitioner roles discussed within this book have been developed in response to this. The culture of service delivery within the NHS is moving swiftly and likewise the practitioners are being expected to adapt their roles accordingly.[6] This has been explicitly described here by those engaged in developing services.

The future holds much uncertainty although the re-election of the present government has enabled policies to continue to be embedded. The whole agenda concerned with Foundation Hospitals and Practice-Based Commissioning will be progressed. The commitment demonstrated at a national level to prescribing rights for non-medical practitioners will also lead to further developments. A report from the BMA conference[7] describes the 'one stop shop' initiative that had been driven by a local GP in Suffolk. This would enable clients to access a variety of services at one location and has implications for partnership agreements between GPs and other groups. This may indeed illustrate the shape of service delivery for the 21st century. Some AHPs are already undertaking training as supplementary prescribers and there are plans for others to be included as indicated by the contributors to this text. Pharmacists will be independent and supplementary prescribers and this may move some services away from GP practices in primary care. There are obvious benefits to pharmacists becoming independent prescribers in relation to their accessibility to the general public. Concerns will continue to be raised in relation to the pharmacy prescription checking procedures and their clinical skills as well as the ethical dimensions relating to prescribing and benefiting financially from the same.

There is increasing engagement with the prescribing process now in secondary care, but also a great deal of uncertainty. The chapters in this book have given an insight into these issues from the practitioners' perspectives. It is clear that if prescribing is going to improve outcomes for patients then it must be developed strategically, with adequate preparation and definition of the role. The DH have recognised this and published an explanatory document for those practitioners less familiar with the concept of prescribing.[8] However, some individuals remain sceptical, especially where they feel that Patient Group Directions (PGD)[9] provide the necessary vehicle for professionals other than medical practitioners to fulfil this role within their practice.

Prescribing in the future may become a mandatory qualification for all nurses. Pre-registration curricula are being developed with this as a consideration. Prescribing for community practitioners has expanded and there continues to be additions to the Nurse Prescribing Formulary for Community Practitioners (NPF).

Although nurse prescribing has become established within the community, particularly where nurses are working in autonomous roles as nurse practitioners, community matrons and practice nurses, there is still ignorance amongst the general public and other health care professionals about the subject. Therefore, the role has yet to be utilised to its full potential. There are also many occasions when the practitioner is unsure of their prescribing rights and responsibilities associated with the evolution of the role.

The availability of medication under General Sales License (GSL) is also undergoing a revolution. The patient can 'self-treat' for such conditions as herpes simplex as Zovirac has been available to purchase for some time. One GP[10] noted how patients with eye infections are now also able to self-medicate by purchasing chloramphenicol previously only available on prescription. From his perspective he recognised the changing nature of consultations at his surgery. He commented that the whole prescribing process has become a minefield. Nurses are increasingly autonomous in assessing patients and completing episodes of care due to their prescribing skills. Pharmacists have also extended their roles in relation to the prescribing of medication. This GP felt aggrieved that those patients who attended surgery with minor ailments that were quick to treat were now being seen by other professionals, leaving him with the more serious and complicated problems that demanded more time to treat! Consequently, appointments were prolonged and patient waiting times were also increased. Ultimately a balance is probably achieved as the GP is required to see fewer patients, freeing up appointments for the more seriously ill. However, this does illustrate the differing expectations of the patient when they visit their doctor. Many people now first consult NHS Direct for advice or surf the Internet for information about their problems before attending the surgery. Access to health care is available at railway stations and walk-in centres as the public demand a more realistic approach for those in full-time occupations unable to adhere to surgery hours. In order to make access to health care more flexible to accommodate the lifestyle of contemporary society it will require all health care practitioners to re-define their roles and working patterns. Prescribing is central to this re-design.

One very real issue is the training of potential prescribers. All students must be supported by a supervisor in practice. Medical practitioners are the only accepted mentors at present but there are problems in identifying doctors willing to supervise students. This is compounded by the fact that there is no financial inducement either. There are also real concerns about the length of the course and the time required away from the practice area. Increasingly, this is being addressed with distance learning and e-learning courses. Whilst these overcome the immediate problems associated with releasing staff to train they place greater pressures on the student and more responsibility on the medical mentor. This is a particular problem in relation to supporting a student isolated from peer support and tutorial supervision.

The future of prescribing is linked to the provision of adequate support and appropriate remuneration. Nurses who have been qualified as prescribers for a few years could also be mentors for those undertaking training. There is anecdotal evidence that this may prove to be a more robust system of mentorship as some nurses have stated that medical mentors are signing them off as competent without the adequate supervision. This engenders a dangerous situation for those in training, as they are having to be assertive with mentors, demanding the appropriate level of supervision. As mentors become more objective (not directly employing the prescribing trainee) this is less likely to be a problem.

The structures must be available at an organisational level to implement this innovation ensuring that the pragmatic elements are fully in place, such as the provision of prescriptions either in paper format or generated electronically. The unavailability of systems for updating patient records has been a particular irritation for clinic-based staff and indeed has been quoted as a reason for community nurses reluctance to embrace this role.

The future is therefore reliant on a whole systems approach which includes workforce planning enabling government targets to be achieved relating to the numbers of practitioners qualified to prescribe. Integral to this approach is the development of information technology systems that provide essential communication across sectors. The national NHS IT project is only being implemented slowly[11] which has implications for prescribing by non-medical staff. The Department of Health's priority is patient safety. Current guidance indicates that independent prescribers should have access to patient records when making prescribing decisions and that records should be updated either at the time of the consultation or within a defined specified time limit.[12]

It is also vital that professionals are enthusiastic to adopt the role and are able to visualise the improvements to the patient experience that will occur. There are increasing opportunities for role development, and prescribing will be an essential skill required to deliver care according to the government's pledge for patients to gain speedier treatment from a more accessible service.

References

1. Latter, S., Maben, J., Myall, M., Courtenay, M., Young, A. and Dunn, N. 'An Evaluation of Extended Formulary Independent Nurse Prescribing: Executive Summary' www.dh.gov.uk/publicationsandstatistics/pressreleases, accessed 29.06.2005.

2. NHS Confederation, British Medical Association. *The New GMS Contract: Investing in General Practice* (London: The NHS Confederation, 2003).

3. Department of Health. *Raising Standards for Patients: New Standards in Out of Hours Care* (London: DH, 2000) www.dh.gov.uk/PolicyAndGuidance/OrganisationPolicy/PrimaryCare/ImplementingOutOf Hours/fs/en, accessed 26.02.06.

4. Department of Health. *Supporting People with Long Term Conditions: Liberating the Talents of Nurses who care for People with Long Term Conditions* (London: DH, 2005) www.dh.gov.uk/PolicyAndGuidance/HealthAndSocialCareTopics/LongTermConditions/LongTermConditionsArticle/fs/en?CONTENT_ID=4128537&chk=hbRPka, accessed 26.02.06.

5. Department of Health. *Our Health Our Care Our Say* (London: DH, 2006) http://www.dh.gov.uk/PolicyAndGuidance/OrganisationPolicy/Modernisation/OurHealthOurCareOurSay/OurHealthBrowsableArticle/fs/en?CONTENT_ID=4130638&MULTIPAGE_ID=5697382&chk=%2BnRboD, accessed 26.02.06.

6. Department of Health. *The Development and Integration of Integrated Governance* (Chief Executive Bulletin: DOH 2004) www.dh.gov.uk/PublicationsAndStatistics, accessed 26.01.06.

7. Carlisle D. 'One stop shop on hold'. *Health Service Journal* (23 June 2005).

8. NHS Moderisation Agency and Department of Health. *Medicine Matters* (London: HMSO, 2005) http://www.dh.gov.uk/assetRoot/04/10/52/26/04105226.pdf, accessed 26.01.06.

9. National Prescribing Centre. *Patient Group Directions. A Practical Guide and Framework of Competencies for all Professionals using Patient Group Directions* (NPC, 2004) www.npc.org.uk, accessed 26.01.06.

10. Copperfield Dr 'It's no more Pills-R-Us'. *Times Body and Soul Supplement*, 16.07.05.

11. Braunold G. 'Site for sore eyes? The IT project struggles to build momentum'. *Health Service Journal* (23.06.2005).

12. Nurse Prescribing Centre (NHS). Connecting Prescribers. www.npc.org.uk, accessed 26.02.06.

Routes of administration for controlled drugs prescribable by nurse independent prescribers for specified indications only

Controlled drug	Indications	Route of administration
Buprenorphine	Palliative care	Transdermal
Chlordiazepoxide hydrochloride	Initial or acute symptoms caused by withdrawal of alcohol where there has been dependency	Oral
Diamorphine hydrochloride	Palliative care Pain relief in suspected myocardial infarction Severe pain after trauma including post-operative pain	Oral and parenteral
Fentanyl	Palliative care	Transdermal
Morphine sulphate	As for diamorphine	Oral, parenteral and rectal
Morphine hydrochloride	As for diamorphine	Rectal
Oxycodone hydrochloride	Palliative care	Oral and parenteral
Diazepam	Palliative care Symptoms caused by withdrawal where there has been dependency	Oral, parenteral and rectal
Lorazepam	Palliative care	Oral and parenteral
Midazolam	Palliative care	parenteral
Codeine phosphate		Oral
Dihydrocodeine tartrate		Oral
Co-phenotrope		Oral

Example Clinical Management Plans

With kind thanks to Simon Sherring and Adrian Rendall for the CMP for treatment of psychosis and to Andy Cole, Community Matron (long-term conditions), Erewash Primary Care Trust for the CMP for treatment of painful peripheral neuropathy.

Please note that these templates are to be used as a guide only and that all Clinical Management Plans need to be individualised and patient specific. Many treatments require blood test monitoring prior to commencement; following dose titration and routinely when prescribed long term. Nurses should ensure that local guidelines relating to monitoring are adhered to. Due to national variations blood monitoring guidance is not included in this book. Some guidance is given in the British National Formulary produced by the British Medical Association and the Royal Pharmaceutical Society of Great Britain.

Clinical Management Plan for Management of Hypertension ≥55 years	
Patient Name:	Patient Medication Sensitivities/allergies:
Patient Identification: (NHS number/ hospital number/date of birth)	Medical History:
Independent Prescriber: Dr Contact Details:	Supplementary Prescriber: Contact details:
Condition to be treated: Hypertension	Aim of Treatment: <ul><li>To reduce systolic BP to <140 mmHg and diastolic BP to <90 mmHg</li><li>In diabetics to reduce systolic BP to <140 mmHg and diastolic BP to <80 mmHg</li><li>To prevent complications secondary to hypertension</li><li>To avoid, or reduce to acceptable levels, side effects from treatment</li></ul>

(Continued)

Preparation	Indication	Dose Schedule	Specific indications for referral back to IP
Thiazide diuretic e.g. Bendroflumethiazide	**Step 1** General first line treatment for older age group	2.5 mg daily (morning)	• Diagnosis in doubt • Unusual blood pressure variability • Elevated serum creatinine or proteinuria • Abnormal sodium or potassium levels • Therapeutic problems (treatment resistance, multiple contraindications or intolerance)
Add ACE Inhibitor e.g. enalapril/lisinopril 2nd Line Ramipril Or Calcium Channel Blocker e.g. amlodopine	**Step 2** if B/P not at required level	2.5 mg once day Titrate according to BNF 1.25 mg once day Titrate according to BNF 5 mg Titrate according to BNF	
Add Calcium Channel Blocker e.g amlodopine Or ACE Inhibitor e.g. enalapril/lisinopril 2nd Line Ramipril	**Step 3** OR others listed in BNF • First line if Thiazide diuretic contra indicated • angina • history of myocardial infarction	5 mg Titrate according to BNF 2.5 mg once day Titrate according to BNF 1.25 mg once day Titrate according to BNF	
Coronary Heart Disease Prevention Aspirin	>50 yrs estimated CHD risk of >15% over 10 yrs with BP controlled to audit standard	75 mg O.D with food	Gastric ulcer, gastric symptoms
LIPID LOWERING THERAPY Simvastatin (contra-indicated in liver disease)	10 yr CHD risk >30% Established atherosclerotic disease	40 mg nocte titrated according to BNF	Abnormal LFTs

Guidelines of protocols supporting Clinical Management Plan

- British Hypertension Society Guidelines 1999
- National Service Framework for Coronary Heart Disease 2000
- Prodigy Guidance Hypertension Updated Sept 2004

Frequency of review and monitoring by: Supplementary Prescriber	Supplementary Prescriber and Independent Prescriber
As Clinically indicated and monthly during treatment titration, at least 6 monthly for review	Date specified (not longer than 1 year)

Process for reporting ADRs:

- Report to Independent prescriber and GP
- Complete adverse reaction form – committee safety of medicines

Shared record to be used by IP and SP:

Lloyd George or computerised patient records

Agreed by independent prescriber(s):	Date	Agreed by Supplementary prescriber(s):	Date	Date agreed with patient/carer:

Clinical Management Plan	Patient Name:
Painful peripheral neuropathy	Date of Birth:
	NHS Number:

Patient Medication Sensitivities/Allergies:	Medical History:
	Type 2 Diabetes Mellitus
	Renal calculi
	Diabetic neuropathy with peripheral nerve involvement

Condition to be treated:	Independent Prescriber:
Diabetic peripheral neuropathy	
Aim of Treatment:	
1. To reduce pain intensity by at least 50%	**Supplementary Prescriber:**
2. To optimise function	
3. Avoid drug interactions and adverse effects	

Medicines that may be prescribed by Supplementary Prescriber:

Preparation Stage 1	Indication	Dose Schedule	Specific Indications for Referral Back to IP
Tricyclic Antidepressant Amitriptyline (unlicensed) *OR*	Failure to relieve pain with paracetamol +/– NSAID alone	10–75 mg once daily	Intolerable side-effects Multiple drug interactions
Anticonvulsant Gabapentin *OR*	Intolerance or failure of amitriptyline to relieve pain	Day 1: 300 mg o.d. Day 2: 300 mg b.d. Day 3: 300 mg t.d.s. then increase by 300 mg daily to max 1.8 g according to response	Failure to improve symptoms or worsening of pain or function Need for specialist referral to pain management centre e.g. higher doses required
Carbamazepine (unlicensed) *AND/OR* *Stage 2*	Failure of gabapentin to improve pain	Initially 100 mg 1–2 times daily, to max of 200 mg 4 times daily	
Opioid Analgesia: Tramadol *OR*	Failure of Stage 1 to improve symptoms	50–100 mg four times daily to maximum of 400 mg daily	
Oxycodone	Failure of tramadol to relieve pain	Initially 5 mg 4–6 hourly to maximum of 400 mg daily	

Guidelines or protocols supporting Clinical Management Plan:

British National Formulary 50 section 6.1.5 (September 2005)

Clinical Management Plan for Management of COPD and Treatment of Acute Exacerbations

Patient Name:	Patient Medication Sensitivities/allergies:

Medical History:

Patient Identification: (NHS number/hospital number/date of birth)

Independent Prescriber:	Supplementary Prescriber:
Dr	Contact details:
Contact Details:	

Condition to be treated:

COPD

Acute Exacerbations of COPD

Aim of Treatment:
- To optimise disease control
- To improve patient: quality of life
- To treat acute exacerbations early and prevent complications

Medicines that may be prescribed by Supplementary Prescriber:

Preparation	Indication	Dose Schedule	Specific indications for referral back to IP
Salbutamol OR Terbutaline inhaler And Ipatroprium Bromide inhaler OR Combivent inhaler	For relief of breathlessness and to aid normal activities For relief of breathlessness and to aid normal activities	200 mcg frequency as specified in BNF, increase frequency during exacerbations 500 mcg frequency as specified in BNF review after 2 months 40–30 mcg frequency as specified in BNF 2 puffs four times daily	Diagnosis is in doubt If supplementary prescriber considers patient may benefit from theophylline treatment If patient needs nebuliser assessment prior to using nebuliser
Volumatic Spacer Inhaler	To increase deposition of drug within the lungs		
Salmeterol OR Formoterol fumarate OR Tiotropium (stop Ipatroprium)	Add in treatment if symptoms not controlled after maximum concentrations of above (discontinue if no improvement after 4 weeks) Where Ipatroprium may not be beneficial. Maintenance treatment	50 mcg twice daily As specified in the BNF As specified in BNF Review benefit after 2 months 18 mcg once daily	Pulse oximetry shows oxygen saturation ≤92% Patient needs oxygen therapy assessment referral Failure to respond to treatment
Beclomethasone Inhaler	Patient has FEV1 ≤ 50% and 2 or more exacerbations in 12 month period needing antibiotics or oral corticosteroids (discontinue if no improvement after 4 weeks)	200–400 mcg twice daily	
Mucolytic therapy Carbocisteine	Chronic cough producing sputum to reduce viscosity	As specified in BNF	

(Continued)

OR Mecysteine hydrochloride	and/or to prevent exacerbations. Continue if effective, review 1 month.	As specified in BNF	
Acute Exacerbation			Lack of response to treatment for acute exacerbation
Oral Prednisolone **AND/OR**	Exacerbation and significant increase in breathlessness	30 mg once daily for 5–14 days	
Amoxycillin **OR**	Exacerbation and sputum more purulent than normal	500 mg three times daily for 5–7 days	
Trimethoprim **OR**	Exacerbation and sputum more purulent than normal	200 mg twice daily for 5–7 days	
Doxycycline	Exacerbation and sputum more purulent than normal	200 mg first day, then 100 mg daily for 10 days	

Guidelines of protocols supporting Clinical Management Plan:

- Local COPD Guidelines, 2004
- NICE Guidelines February 2004
- BNF March 2006
- Prodigy Guidance – COPD Last revised July 2006

Frequency of review and monitoring by:

Supplementary Prescriber	Supplementary Prescriber and Independent Prescriber
As Clinically indicated by response but at least 6 monthly	Date specified no longer than 1 year

Process for reporting ADRs:

- Report to Independent prescriber and GP
- Complete adverse reaction form – committee safety of medicines

Shared record to be used by IP and SP:

Lloyd George or computerised patient records

Agreed by independent prescriber(s):	Date	Agreed by Supplementary prescriber(s):	Date	Date agreed with patient/carer:

Clinical Management Plan for Type 2 Diabetes	
Patient Name:	**Patient Medication Sensitivities/allergies:**
	Medical History:
Patient Identification: (NHS number/ hospital number/date of birth)	
Independent Prescriber: Dr **Contact Details:**	**Supplementary Prescriber:** **Contact details:**
Condition to be treated: Type 2 Diabetes	**Aim of Treatment:** • To optimise glycaemic control • To educate and support patient in diabetes care • Prevention/delay progression of microvascular and macrovascular complications

Medicines that may be prescribed by Supplementary Prescriber:			
Preparation	**Indication**	**Dose Schedule**	**Specific indications for referral back to IP**
Oral hypoglycaemics **Biguanide:** Metformin 500 mg (contra-indicated in renal impairment, ketoacidosis)	First line treatment unless contra-indicated	Titrate as specified in BNF	If optimal control is not achieved. If there is an adverse drug reaction If SP feels patient might benefit from thiazolinediones or insulin
Sulphonylureas: Gliclazide 80 mg (contra-indicated in severe hepatic & renal impairment	Add in treatment in combination with metformin if clinically indicated	40 mg OD, increase as required as specified in BNF 1 to 3 monthly to achieve glucose control or until maximum tolerated dose. As specified in BNF	Worsening renal or hepatic function Presence of microalbuminuria or proteinuria – for consideration of ACE inhibitors
Hypostop gel/ glucagon injection	As treatment for hypoglycaemia		

Guidelines of protocols supporting Clinical Management Plan:
• NICE Guidelines September 2002
• Local Guidelines on the Management of Diabetes May 2004
• NICE guidance on Rosiglitazone and Pioglitazone
• BNF Sept. 2004

Frequency of review and monitoring by:
Monitoring of urine/blood glucose testing and follow-up by telephone or in person by:

Supplementary Prescriber	Supplementary prescriber and independent prescriber
At least weekly during dose titration and treatment changes and then as clinically indicated	Date specified no longer than 12 months

Process for reporting ADRs:
• Report to Independent prescriber and GP
• Complete adverse reaction form – committee safety of medicines

Shared record to be used by IP and SP:
Paper Lloyd George and computerised patient records

Agreed by independent prescriber(s):	Date	Agreed by Supplementary prescriber(s):	Date	Date agreed with patient/carer:

Clinical Management Plan for Management of Heart Failure	
Patient Name: **Patient Identification: (NHS number/hospital number/date of birth)**	**Patient Medication Sensitivities/allergies:** **Medical History:**
Independent Prescriber: Dr **Contact Details:**	**Supplementary Prescriber:** **Contact details:**
Condition to be treated: Heart Failure due to Left Ventricular Systolic Dysfunction	**Aim of Treatment:** • To improve/reduce symptoms associated with heart failure • To improve quality of life • To prevent complications secondary to heart failure • To avoid, or reduce to acceptable levels, side effects from treatment

Medicines that may be prescribed by Supplementary Prescriber:

Preparation	Indication	Dose Schedule	Specific indications for referral back to IP
ACE Inhibitor e.g. enalapril	**Step 1** General first line treatment	2.5 mg daily (morning) titrate to maximum tolerated dose for control of symptoms (maximum 40 mg) in two divided doses	• Diagnosis in doubt • Unusual blood pressure variability systolic blood pressure below 90 mm/Hg • Elevated serum creatinine 30% above patient's usual • Therapeutic problems (treatment resistance, multiple contraindications or intolerance) • Clinical indication for higher dose of loop diuretic • Clinical indication for use of spironolactone
Loop Diuretic Furosemide Or Bumetanide	Oedema present	40 mg O.D to maximum of 120 mg in one or two divided doses 1–2 mg in one or two divided doses	
Add Beta Blocker e.g. Bisoprolol	**Step 2** Symptoms not controlled	1.25 mg once daily and titrate according to BNF to maximum of 10 mg	

Guidelines of protocols supporting Clinical Management Plan:

• NICE Guideline for Chronic Heart Failure 2003
• Prodigy Guidance Hypertension Updated June 2004
• Local guidelines 2006

Frequency of review and monitoring by:	
Supplementary Prescriber	Supplementary Prescriber and Independent Prescriber
As Clinically indicated during treatment titration, at least 6 monthly for review	Date to be included no longer than 1 year

Process for reporting ADRs:

• Report to Independent prescriber and GP
• Complete adverse reaction form – committee safety of medicines

Shared record to be used by IP and SP:

Lloyd George or computerised patient records

Agreed by independent prescriber(s):	Date	Agreed by Supplementary prescriber(s):	Date	Date agreed with patient/carer:

Name of Patient:	Patient medication sensitivities/allergies:

Patient identification e.g. ID number, date of birth

Address of Patient:

Current Medication: Olanzapine 4 mg daily	Medical History:

Independent Prescriber(s): Consultant psychiatrist (Name) Contact details: (tel/email/address)	Supplementary Prescriber(s): Mental Health Nurse (Name) Contact details: (tel/email/address)

Condition(s) to be treated: Psychosis	Aim of Treatment: Control psychotic episodes

Medicines that may be prescribed by Supplementary Prescriber:

Preparation	Indication	Dose Schedule	Specific indications for referral back to independent prescriber
Respiradone	Psychosis	Increase by 1 mg increments to a total of 8 mg	Symptoms unresponsive after increasing dose to 8 mg New side effects reported by patient If change of medication were indicated

Guidelines or protocols supporting Clinical Management Plan:
BNF, September 2005
NICE Guidelines for schizophrenia
Local Guidelines/policies, 2005

(Continued)

Frequency of review and monitoring by:	
Supplementary Prescriber: Twice weekly or more often if indicated	**Supplementary Prescriber and Independent Prescriber:** 3 to 6 monthly (Care Programme Approach) NB Date will be specified

Process for reporting ADRs:
Yellow Card
Patient Notes

Shared record to be used by Independent and Supplementary prescriber:
Computerised clinical notes system
Letter to patient's GP

Agreed by Independent Prescriber(s) Sign:	Date	Agreed by Supplementary Prescriber(s) Sign:	Date	Agreed with patient/carer:
				Name: Date:

Appendix 3

The Twelve Principles of Writing a Prescription

1. Prescriptions should be written legibly in ink.
2. Should be dated, with the full name and address of the patient and should be signed in ink by the prescriber.
3. It is a legal requirement when prescribing prescription only medicines (POMs) for the age to be stated in children under 12 years. It preferably should be stated on all occasions.
4. The unnecessary use of decimal points should be avoided for example 3 mg not 3.0 mg.
5. Micrograms, nanograms and units should not be abbreviated.
6. Millilitre should be used rather than cubic centimetre.
7. Dose and frequency should be stated. If a preparation can be taken 'as required' a minimum dose interval should be specified.
8. The names of medicines and preparations should be written clearly and not abbreviated, using approved and generic names only.
9. The symbol NP on NHS forms should be deleted if it is required that the name of the preparation should not appear on the label.
10. The quantity to be supplied should be stated and the number of days treatment is required.
11. Although directions should be in English without abbreviation it is recognised that some Latin abbreviations are used.
12. When prescribing unlicensed medicines the patient or carer should be told that the product does not have marketing authorisation.

Source: British National Formulary.

Clinical Management Plan Template

TEMPLATE CMP 1 (Blank): For teams that have full co-terminus access to patient records

Name of Patient:		Patient medication sensitivities/allergies:	
Patient identification e.g. ID number, date of birth:			
Independent Prescriber(s):		Supplementary Prescriber(s)	
Condition(s) to be treated		Aim of treatment	
Medicines that may be prescribed by SP:			
Preparation	Indication	Dose schedule	Specific indications for referral back to the IP
Guidelines or protocols supporting Clinical Management Plan:			
Frequency of review and monitoring by:			
Supplementary prescriber	Supplementary prescriber and independent prescriber		
Process for reporting ADRs:			
Shared record to be used by IP and SP:			

Agreed by independent prescriber(s)	Date	Agreed by supplementary prescriber(s)	Date	Date agreed with patient/carer

TEMPLATE CMP 2 (Blank): For teams where the SP does not have co-terminus access to the medical record

Name of Patient:	Patient medication sensitivities/allergies:
Patient identification e.g. ID number, date of birth:	
Current medication:	Medical history:
Independent Prescriber(s): Contact details: [tel/email/address]	Supplementary prescriber(s): Contact details: [tel/email/address]
Condition(s) to be treated:	Aim of treatment:

Medicines that my be prescribed by SP:

Preparation	Indication	Dose schedule	Specific indications for referral back to the IP

Guidelines or protocols supporting Clinical Management Plan:

Frequency of review and monitoring by:

Supplementary prescriber	Supplementary prescriber and independent prescriber

Process for reporting ADRs:

Shared record to be used by IP and SP:

Agreed by independent prescriber(s):	Date	Agreed by supplementary prescriber(s):	Date	Date agreed with patient/carer

Source: DH, Clinical Management Plans. Used with kind permission. www.dh.gov.uk/assetRoot/04/06/81/28/04068428.rtf accessed 20 April 2006.

Index